To be effective, the yoga postures (asanas) described and illustrated in this book require musical elixirs, free with purchase of the book. To obtain your copy of this music, two options are offered:

A. To download the music, go to www.yogaofillumination.com;

B. To obtain the physical CDs, you may either:

    a. email sj@almine.net, providing your name and mailing address, or

    b. call toll-free 877-552-5646 or 614-354-2071.

The effectiveness of this modality is heightened by at least 15 minutes of meditation on a verse from The Poetry of Dreaming, accompanied by music from the elixirs, prior to beginning the yoga.

IRASH SATVA
YOGA

Restoring the Abundant Life

Almine

The Yoga to Open the Gates of
Abundant Resources

Published by Spiritual Journeys LLC

Copyright 2010
MAB 998 Megatrust

By Almine
Spritual Journeys LLC
P.O. Box 300
Newport, Oregon 97365

Cover Illustration—Dorian Dyer
www.visionheartart.com

Cover Layout—Rogier Chardet
Layout—Ariel Frailich

Manufactured in the United States of America

ISBN 978-1-934070-95-6

Contents

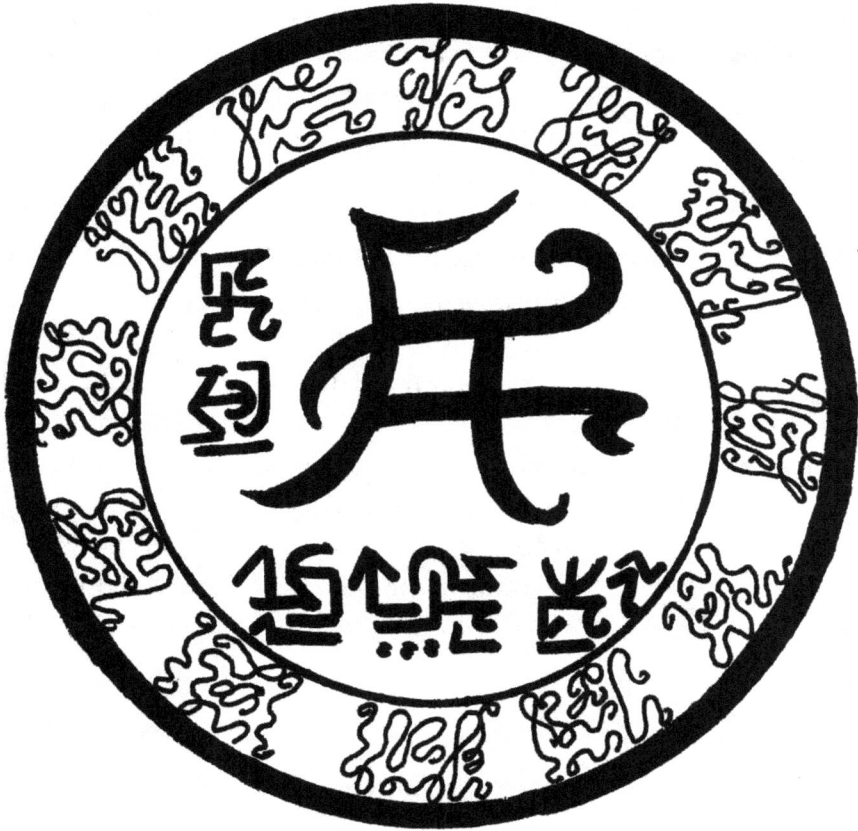

Irash Satva Yoga
The Song of Life Yoga

"What a priceless experience to be able to catch a glimpse into one of the most remarkable lives of our time..."
— H.E. Ambassador Armen Sarkissian,
Former Prime Minister of the Republic of Armenia,
Astro-physicist, Cambridge University, U.K.

"I'm really impressed with Almine and the integrity of her revelations. My respect for her is immense and I hope that others will find as much value in her teaching as I have."
— Dr. Fred Bell, Former NASA Scientist

"The information she delivers to humanity is of the highest clarity. She is fully deserving of her reputation as the leading mystic of our age."
— Zbigniew Ostas, Ph.D. Quantum Medicine,
Somatidian Orthobiology, Canada and Poland

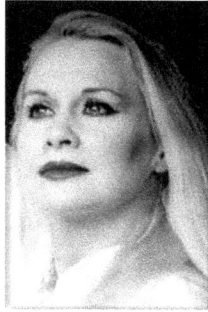

About the Author

Almine is widely regarded as the leading mystic of our time. Author of 11 books and originator of the globally acclaimed healing modality, Belvaspata; she shares her wisdom with a rapidly growing worldwide audience on a daily basis. (See www.alminediary.com, www.facebook.com/SeersWisdom and www.twitter.com/alminewisdom). Her profound wisdom and unparalleled inter-dimensional abilities have been acclaimed by scientists and students alike.

"When we live in the moment, we live in the place of power, aligned with eternal time and the intent of the Infinite. Our will becomes blended with that of the Divine."

—Almine

Note: Almine has for many years translated tablets and records from inter-dimensional sources to reveal sacred information previously unavailable to humanity. It is only in the last months of 2009 that some of her students have been able to obtain photographic evidence of the existence of these materials. See the following pages for examples of inter-dimensional photos of tablets previously translated by her.

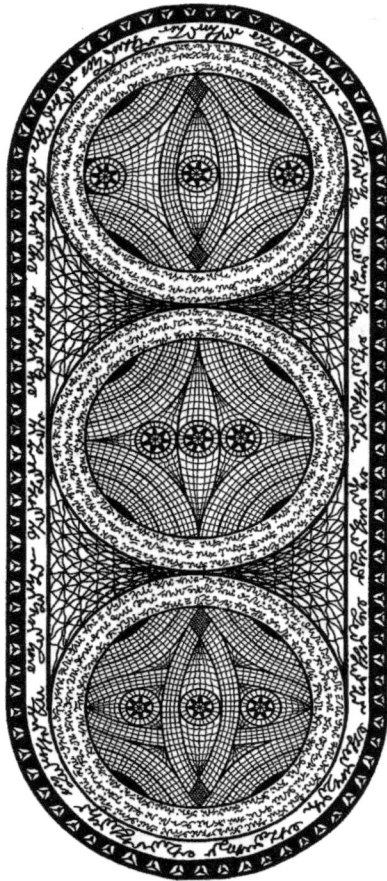

Tablets drawn and translated by Almine
months before they were photographed.

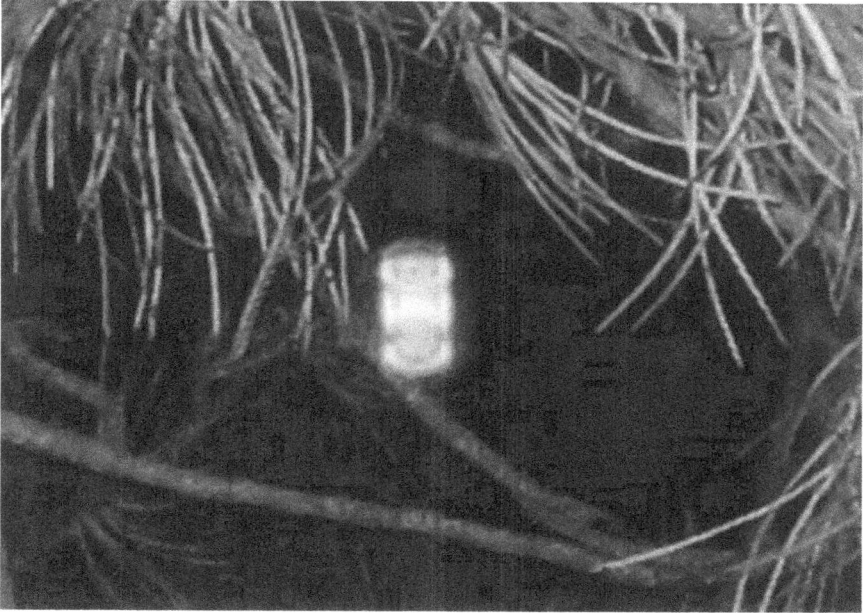
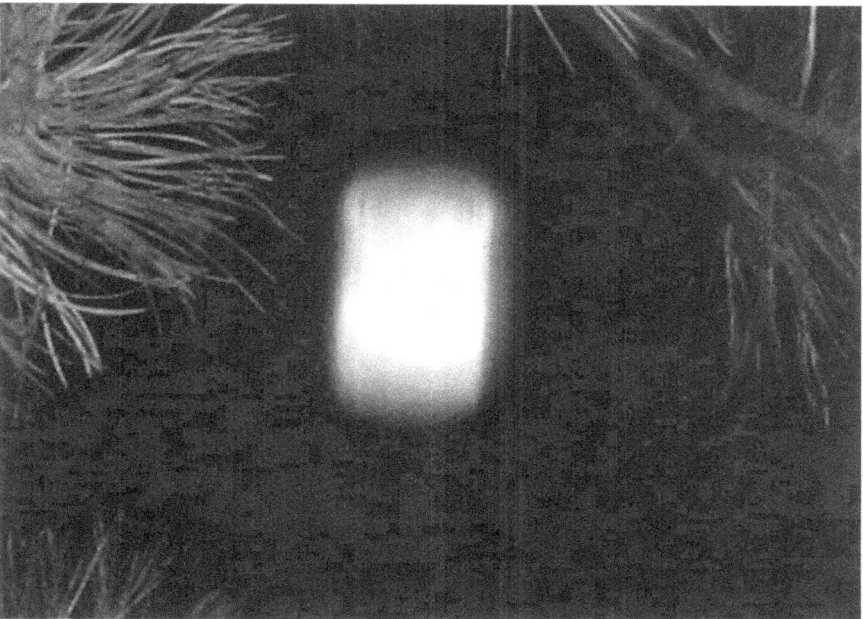

Photos taken by Barbara Rotzoll, 2009 (angelbarbara.com)

Introduction

In its original state, the physical form was meant to be self-purifying, self-regenerating and self-transfiguring. Being created, it was not real or eternal but could, through pristine living and total surrender, open gates in the body that would allow the Real to permeate and indefinitely sustain it.

In most, the 144 cardinal gates contain debris from programming, resistance to life and the belief systems generated by an illusory reality. This yoga, kept by the Angelic Kingdom since the dawn of existence, is called in the angelic language "Michpa uresvi minavech", or 'The source of the rivers of life.' It is the ancient parent of later forms of bodily yogas and works with the alchemy of sound.

Once mastered, it can be taught to others[1] with the condition that Almine is credited as its physical originator. The angelic records are clear that its true source is the 'Arachve Aranat', the embodiment of the One Life.

Every cardinal gate has an associated concept of abundant life and those 144 concepts should be studied. If teaching a class, spend a half-hour studying them in depth and one hour doing the physical yoga. Each gate has a name and because it has a beneficial frequency the instructor can, if desired, say the names while the posture is maintained.

---

1 It can be taught to children as well as adults.

BIRAKLET KANESH IRASH SATVA
Opening to the Song of Life

Serenachvi harish-sat eklet nunatras haravut
Prives u-eres areskava uknech ehere-varastat
Biset uras para bi-uklet arsatvi-i-unech bersta
Uklech miriheshavat ustet pirech ukletvi verusat
Mi-uhes pire vesvi usklu-anat michtret ba-rusta

TRANSLATION OF THE
BIRAKLET KANESH IRASH SATVA

1. In those who resist life, the cellular nucleus is closed.
2. One hundred and forty-four cardinal gates in the body exist.
3. When these are open, the cells start to change.
4. The nucleus becomes irregular and enlarged.
5. The spiritualized cells produce immortality.

Understanding the Practices

Understanding Irash Satva Yoga

THE DIVINE PURPOSE OF THIS YOGA

The body holds 144 points that, when fully opened, act as sluices for the supply of infinite resources. They become the channels between the beginningless reality of existence and the holographic, illusory reality of form. In Ascended Masters, many of these points or gateways are open, prolonging vibrant life for thousands of years.[2]

By becoming gateways for the resources of the Infinite, consciousness in Cosmic Life is raised. This leaves the cosmos in the yogi's debt and according to the law of compensation that debt must be repaid. The yogi's consciousness is raised as a consequence.

The Breathing Techniques

The breaths are slowly drawn in and then slowly released, like a prolonged sigh. Breathe in through the nose, out through the mouth. In this way birth trauma is released which is a major contributory factor to blockage in the cardinal gates. This breathing method also releases the debris of past life experience.

Normal, deep, nose breathing helps to release the tension of linear time and daily stress, as well as that produced by belief systems and identity. Alternating these breathing methods from one complete session to the next is helpful (do not vary breathing methods during one session of 26 postures).[3]

---

2 See The Science of Immortality and Incorruptibility on www.alchemyandmysticism.com
3 The yoga is best done in a comfortably warm temperature.

The Pressure and Postures

The body has traditionally been a tyrant. During the yoga session it is schooled to become disciplined. There are a few general techniques to be utilized throughout sessions. When your palms are held together, exert gentle but firm pressure. Activate pressure points with the same technique. Tapping is likewise to be gentle but firm. The points down the side of the ribcage are firmly tapped, however. Drink plenty of water after a session.

The Mystical Elixirs

The term 'elixir' when applied to music[4] indicates that the alchemical knowledge of the potencies of frequencies has been applied to produce a sound healing that eliminates illusion. DO NOT USE MUSIC OTHER THAN THE 26 SOUND ELIXIRS DESIGNED FOR THIS YOGA.

The use of black (subliminal) frequencies, together with an equal amount of white frequencies, balances them and cancels out illusion. This balance has been employed in the creation of the elixir music, which was channeled from the angelic realms.

The information in this book is not intended to diagnose illness or to constitute medical advice or treatment. All healing takes place within self. Please follow all regulatory guidelines of your specific municipality in terms of assisting and working with others, even with their express consent. A physician should be consulted for any necessary medical attention.

Pregnant or health conditions: Consult with your physician or other qualified health provider with any questions you may have regarding pregnancy or any specific medical conditions prior to the start of any exercise program.

---

4 See www.angelsoundhealing.com

KASHAR-AVI BIRESAT IRASH SATVA YOGA
The sacred origins of Irash Satva Yoga

Usutra aklechbi hesetru mirusat aklevish estalvi
Ninubich esta-brivech heleshta miruvetiklet
Nanas bri-ues plava ninech iselklava unes
Bri-es paravat usute blavech uvasp manech
Kanes esavit uskalvi minech harut uvesbi

TRANSLATION OF
KASHAR-AVI BIRESAT IRASH SATVA YOGA

1. In the time of the dream, when form began,
2. Self-sustenance was part of existence.
3. Eternal resources entered the body through gates.
4. When the gates became blocked, polarity became a substitute energy source.
5. In the yoga of Oneness shall they open to the Eternal Supply.

The Gift of the Angels

IRASH SATVA YOGA

Discord within humanity has come to be
From pollution, genetics have corrupted been
Vaccines and hostile waveforms unseen
Have caused discord that must be cleaned

A Yoga we bring, of form and frequency
To remove toxins and calcifications caused by
the beliefs of mind
The frequencies of higher life man had before
The new Song of Life within humanity to restore

How to do the Yoga

The Yoga to Restore the Harmonious Frequencies of Man

IRASH SATVA YOGA

Note: All 24 sound elixirs of the Hidden Kingdoms will be used. The two elixirs of Klanivik are inserted after the 12th and 25th elixirs of the Hidden Kingdoms. These are not only in a much faster tempo (at variance with the meditative tempo of the 24 Hidden Kingdoms elixirs) but are each about six minutes long. The specific yoga positions given for that part of the music need to be held for their duration.

The elixirs facilitate the removal of toxins from the gateways located at each position; the first 12 from the masculine, pro-active gateways and the last 12 from the feminine/receptive ones. They are catalysts for stimulating the blood and lymph flow and liver function.

––––––––––––

There are 26 yoga postures to be done as the 26 elixirs are played, that can release toxins from the body. Each posture is held during the entire duration of its corresponding elixir. Gradually ease into the postures if you are not athletically active. At no time should you do more than a comfortable gentle stretch. You and the room should be comfortably warm to stimulate the release of toxins.

This Posture to Sound yoga is called Irash Satva Yoga – the frequency body yoga.

The Names of the Postures Used in the Ancient Technique of Irash Satva

The Stretching Postures – Asaf-pirehut

1. Ignati Rururet
2. Bligavesh
3. Bligavesh Iglat
4. Bligavesh Uret
5. Nisavi Vishnatet
6. Harasvu Isabi
7. Kunimani
8. Ra-vanavish
9. Siti-vanavish
10. Rutga-vanavish
11. Knanani-usubetvi
12. Kasabi-usubetvi[5]
13. Kanatchi-esanum (the catalyst)

The Tapping Postures – Nananani-usep

14. Kushana-paarsi
15. Nechsu-varish
16. Aasabi Plishet
17. Kanachvu
18. Nasaar Isalvu
19. Saru Bishar
20. Saru Eleshar
21. Nasu Anagu
22. Kaarsh-haras
23. Nistu Arana

---

5 The last of the masculine postures.

24. Kivistu Branesh

The Pressure Postures – Kuhulu-satvi
25. Agnanut-havi[6]
26. Bru-ak-nespahu (the catalyst)

---

6 The last of the feminine postures.

The 26 Postures

(Use a yoga mat if possible)

THE STRETCHING POSTURES – ASAF-PIREHUT

1. Ignati Rururet

While on your knees, raise your arms above your head in a gentle stretch. Relax back and sit on your heels. Bend forward, keeping your arms in their outstretched position as though bending as low as you can go to a king. Keep your hips back on your heels. Relax.

Note: If at any time your position causes dizziness, lie down on your mat.

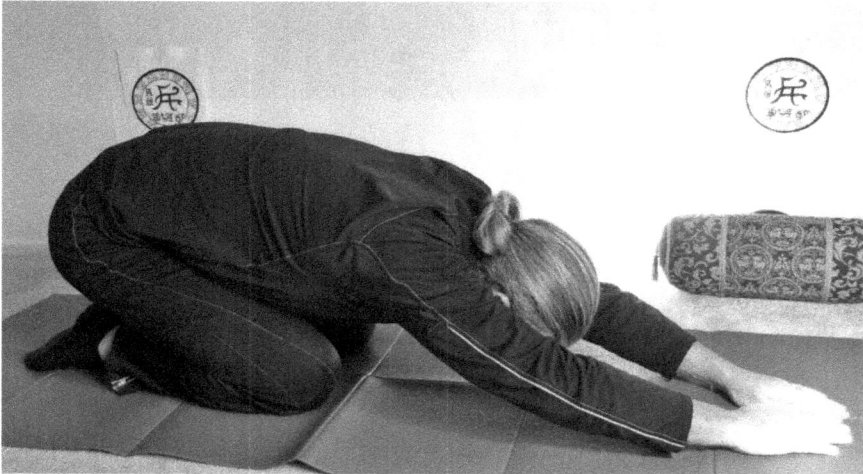

2. Bligavesh

Lie flat on your back with your knees bent as far towards your chest as possible with comfort. Hug your knees with both arms and clasp your hands together, holding your knee position in place.

(For both postures 3 and 4, the use of a pillow may be more comfortable for some.)

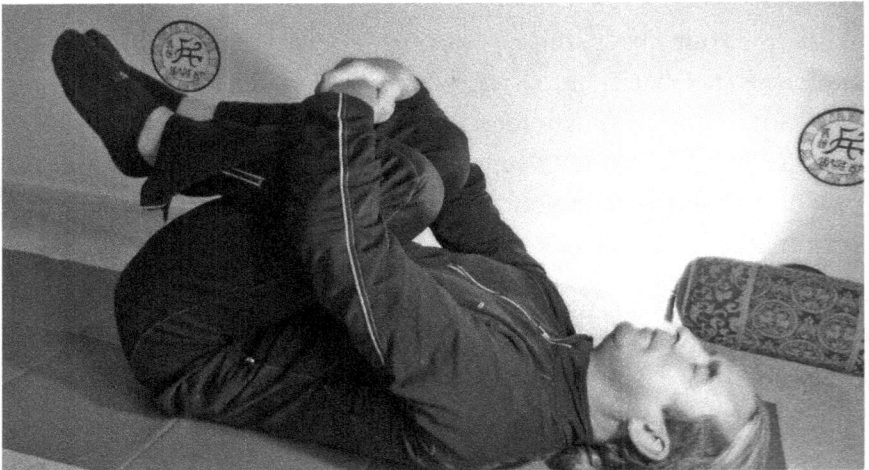

3. Bligavesh Iglat

Do the exact same posture as that used in the second Bligavesh posture, except while lying on your left side. If it is not comfortable to rest the left side of your body on the mat during this posture, brace the legs by placing a pillow under them; you may also use a small pillow under your head.

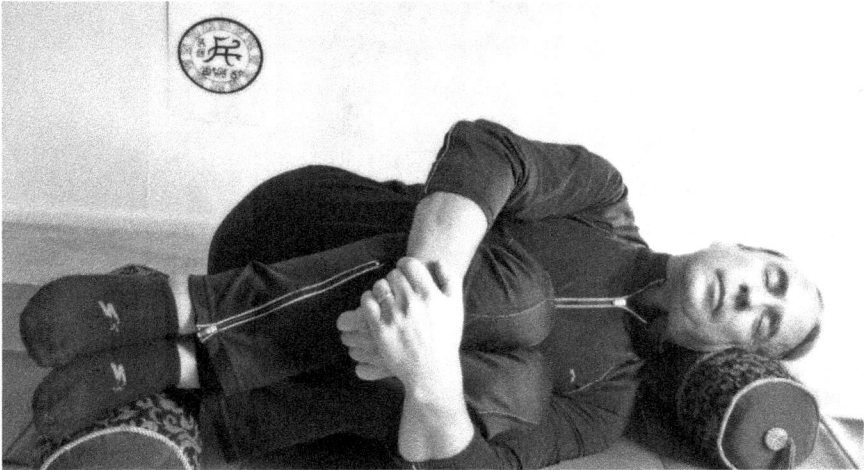

4. Bligavesh Uret

Repeat the Bligavesh Iglat posture, but lie on your right side. (Demonstration of the posture without pillows.)

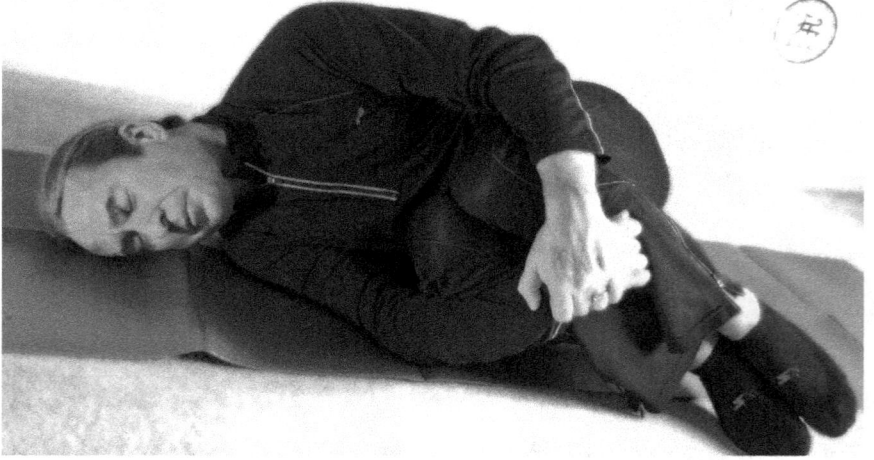

5. Nisavi Vishnatet

Lie on your back with your arms outstretched to the side. Keeping your feet a shoulder-width apart, raise your knees by bringing the feet towards your body (the feet will be where your knees used to be when the legs were flat). Keep the buttocks clenched for the duration of the elixir.

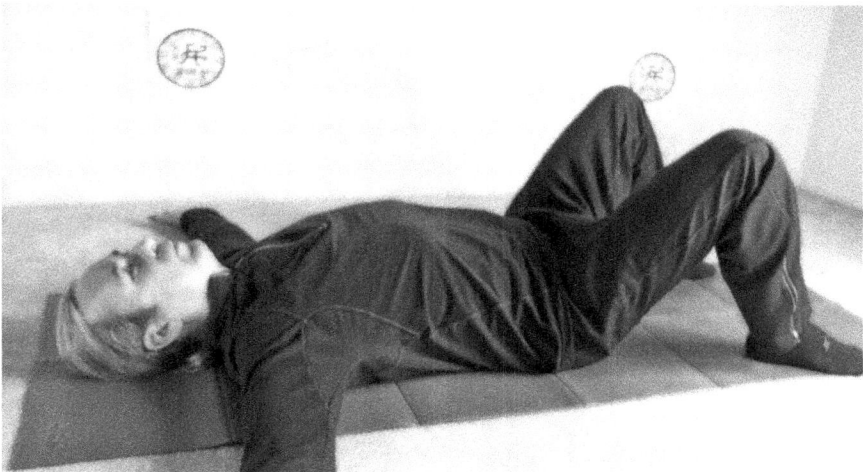

6. Harasvu Isabi

In the exact same posture as the Nisavi Vishnatet in No. 5, raise the buttocks off the floor and hold. A pillow may be placed underneath the hips to support their raised position.

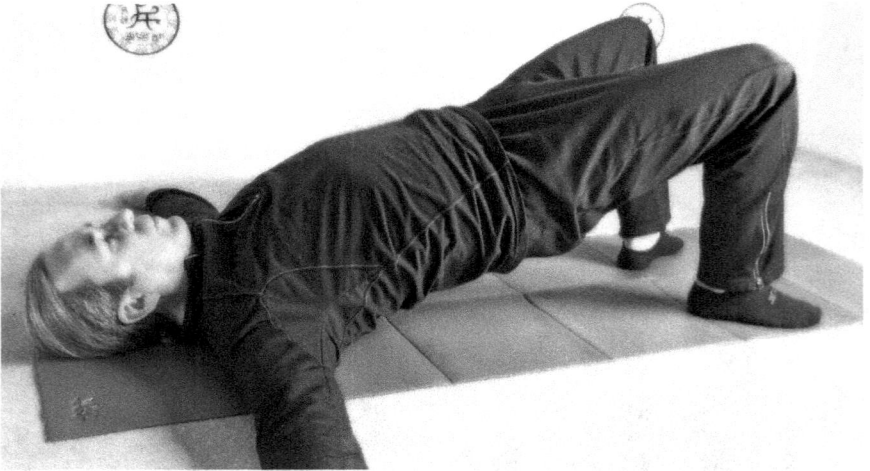

7. Kunimani

Sit cross-legged with the spine straight. If you are not able to cross your legs, have the soles of your feet touch each other. Clasp your hands over your solar plexus, elbows extended outward to the side. Take deep, rhythmic breaths.

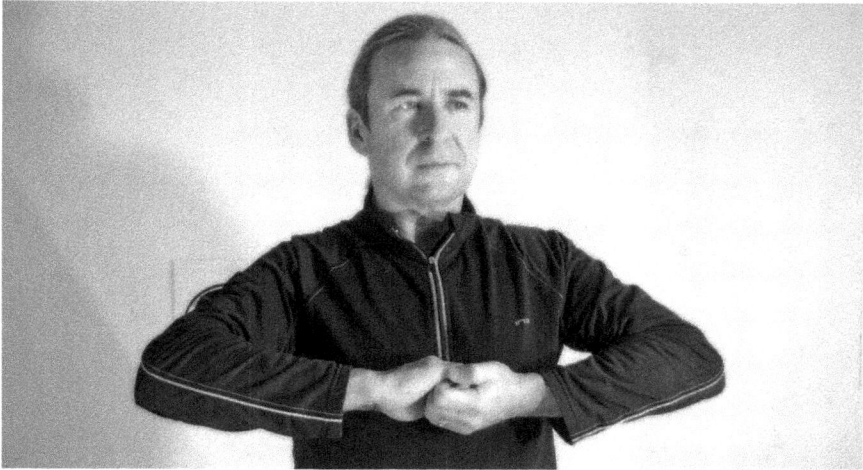

8. Ra-vanavish

Keep the same posture as in No. 7, drop your clasped hands into your lap. Unclasp them and let them lie in a relaxed position on your thighs. Bend the pinkies (little fingers) and ring ringers towards the palm keeping the other fingers outstretched. Drop your head forward in a gentle stretch onto your chest.

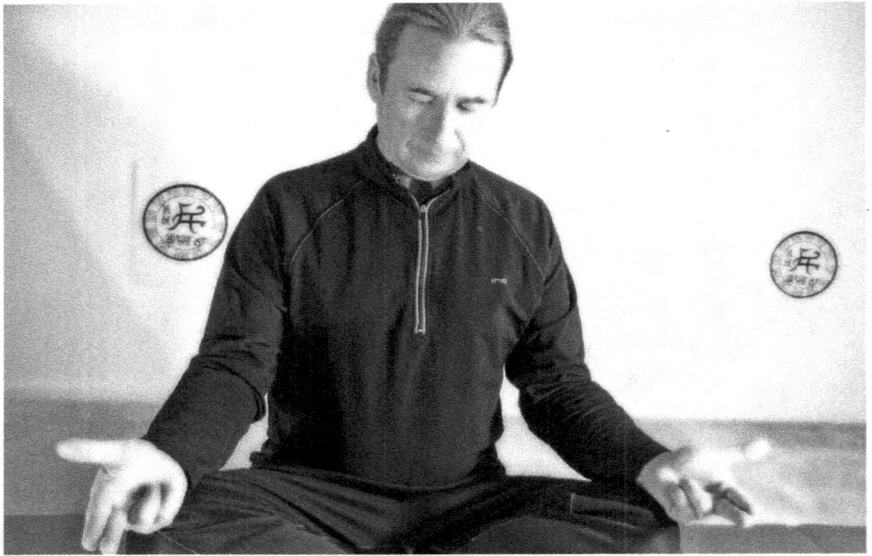

9. Siti-vanavish

Repeat the same posture as for Ra-vanavish in No. 8, but move the head as far left as is comfortable, with the chin on the left shoulder (do not raise the shoulder, just drop the chin to achieve a comfortable gentle stretch).

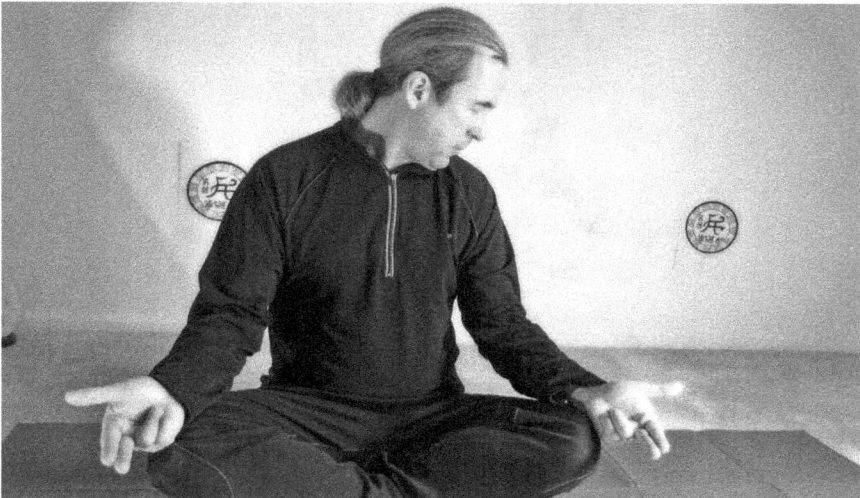

10. Rutga-vanavish
Repeat No. 9, but on the right side, chin towards the right shoulder.

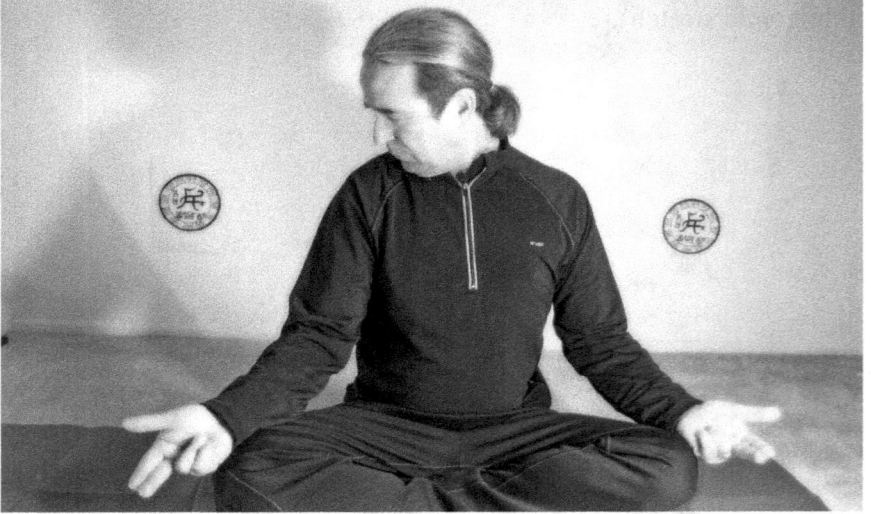

11. Knanani-usubetvi

Stay in the same cross-legged position (or with soles of feet together) as before, clasp your hands together over the sternum, elbows extended towards the side. Raise your chin and keep your head facing forward as you rotate from the waist to the left. Your head and lower body will be facing forward; your upper torso will be rotated to the left.

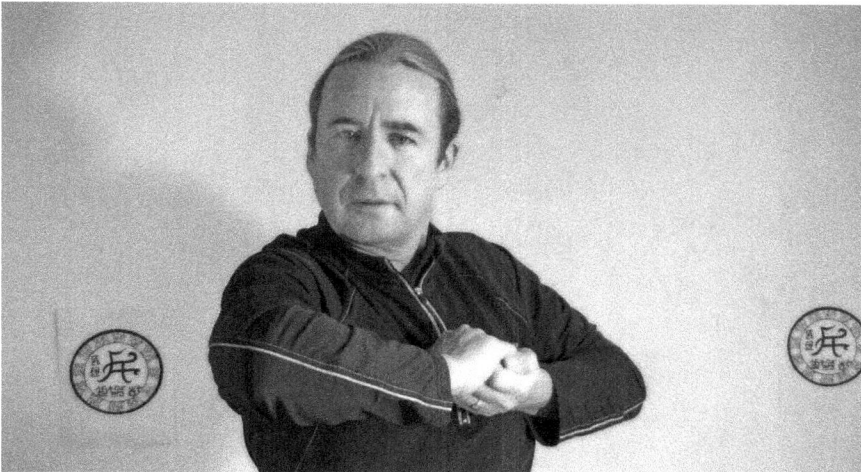

12. Kasabi-usubetvi

Repeat No. 11, Knanani-usubetvi, but rotate the upper torso to the right.

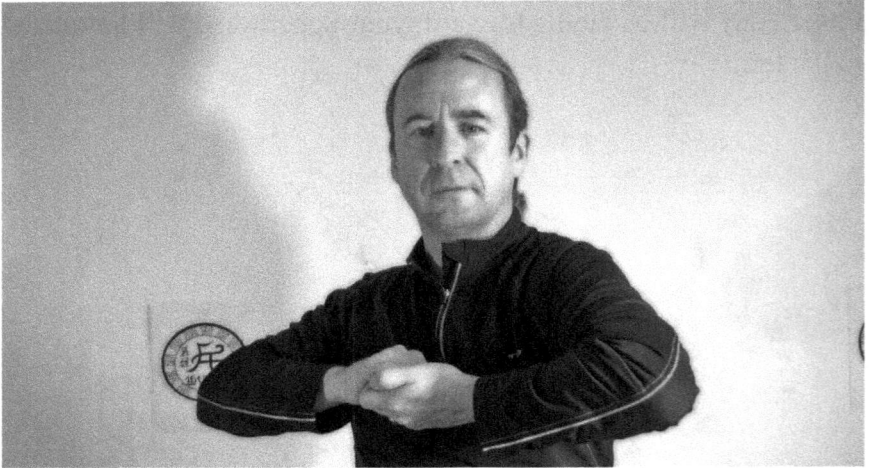

13. Kanatchi-esanum

Lying flat on your back, arms outstretched above your head, bend the elbows slightly with palms together, resting your arms comfortably on the mat. Bend your knees slightly outward to place the soles of your feet together. Your legs should be as flat on the mat as possible. Place a pillow under the knees for comfort if needed.

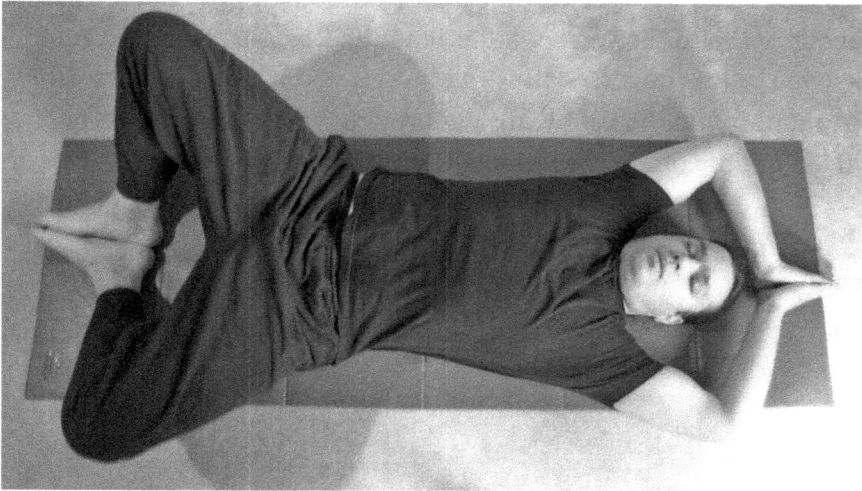

THE TAPPING POSITIONS – NANANANI-USEP

14. Kushana-paarsi

This position requires that you sit with the soles of the feet together (use a pillow under the knees if it is more comfortable) and your spine straight. With the thumbs over the bent small and ring fingers of both hands, extend your middle and index fingers, keeping them close together. Tap twice on each of the 9 pressure points, starting about 1-1.5" directly above the inner end of the eyebrow, directly above the tear duct (see illustration). Use both hands simultaneously, tapping lightly, following the brow bone's contours and ending in the middle of the cheekbone. Repeat for the duration of the elixir.

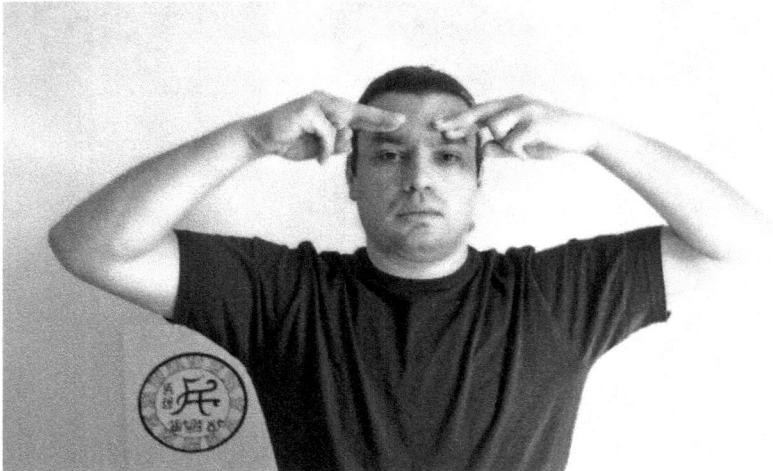

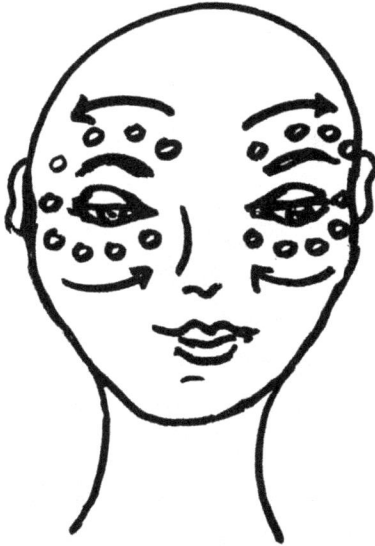

Kushana-paarsi

Tap twice on each point, repeat,
but start each repetition above the brow.

15. Nechsu-varish

With the same hand and body position as used in No. 14, tap twice on the eight points illustrated. Using both hands simultaneously, start on the temple point (called Kaanish, which means 'holy') directly out from the outer corners of the eyes. Tap lightly twice on each point, moving in an arch around the ears and ending just below the skull behind the ears. Repeat, always moving in the same direction.

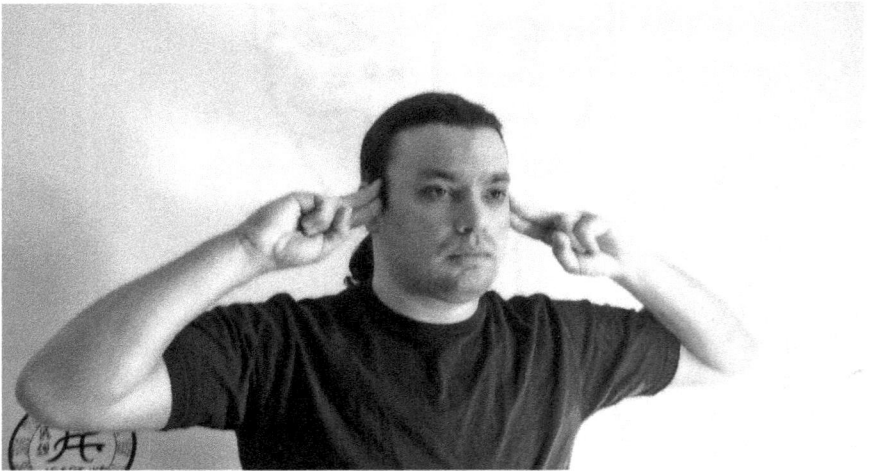

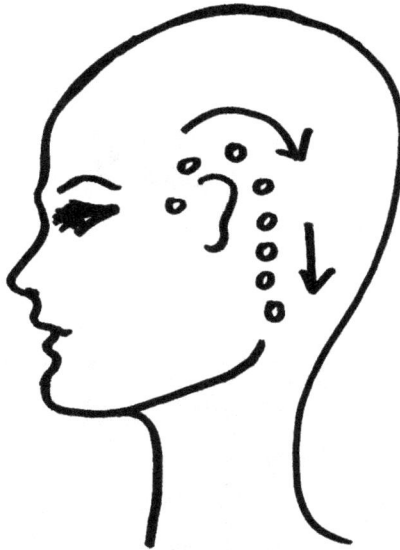

Nechsu-varish

There are eight points. The first point is directly above
the cheekbone. Arch around the ear, ending just below the skull. Always repeat in the same direction.

16. Aasabi Plishet

Beginning directly behind the earlobes, using the same hand and body postures as in Nos. 14 & 15, tap twice on each of the seven points, always repeating in the same direction as illustrated. Use both hand simultaneously.

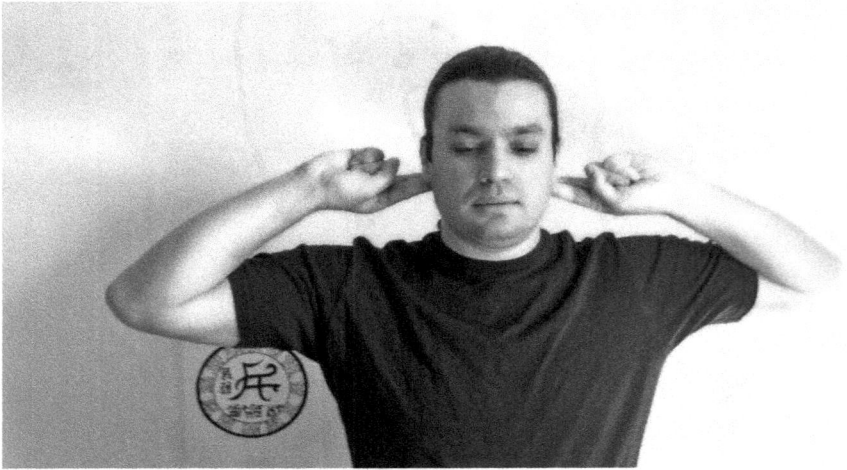

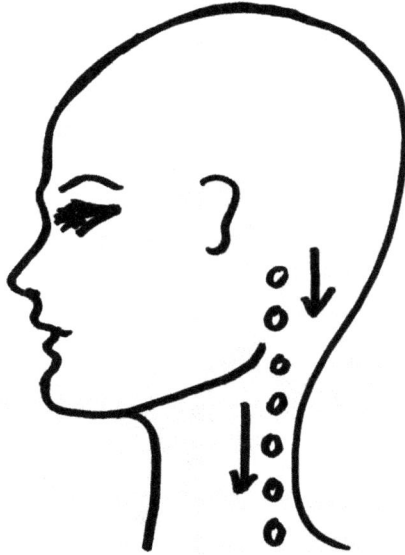

Aasabi Plishet

There are seven points. Start behind the earlobes,
moving along the front of the neck muscles. End at
the point where the neck and shoulders meet.

17. Kanachvu

This uses the same hand and body postures as those preceding. There are six tapping points; each is to be tapped twice. The hands will be moving in opposite directions, starting on the sternum in the middle of the chest. The starting point is 2" below the hollow of the throat at the base of the neck.

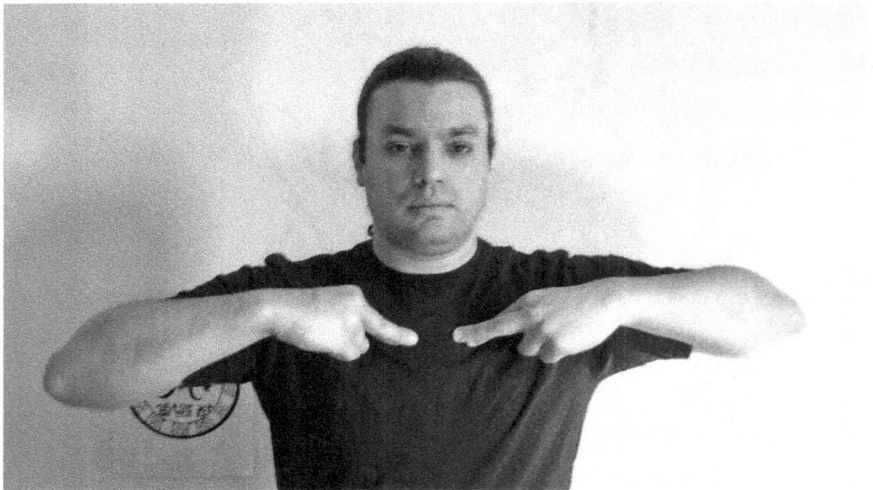

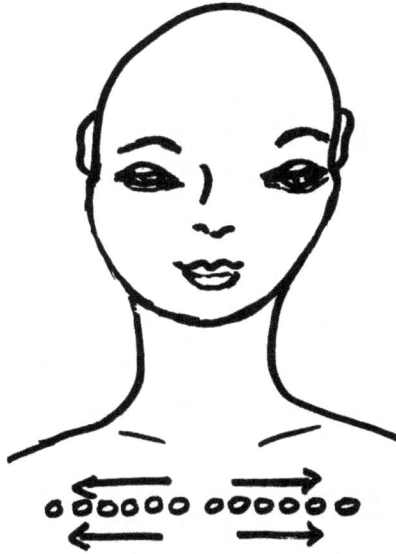

Kanachvu

Repeat all tapping postures for the duration of their
corresponding elixir. Always tap from the sternum
outwards — the hands will be moving in opposite
directions.

18. Nasaar Isalvu

Use the same postures and procedures as in No. 17 and start from the same point, 2" below the hollow of the throat. With the index fingers 1" apart, tap five points downward. Repeat in the same direction, always moving toward the heart.

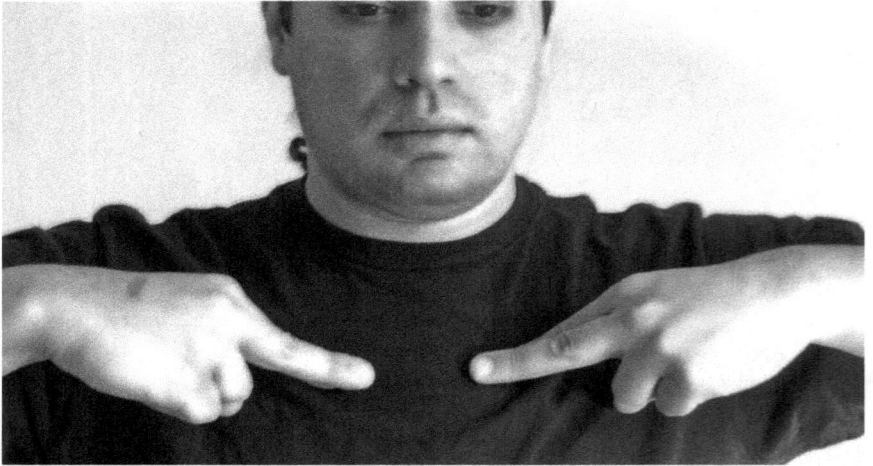

19. Saru Bishar

Remain in the same seated position, raise your left arm as high as it can go in a comfortable stretch. From the waist, lean to the right until there is a stretch down the left side of the torso. Using the two fingers of the right hand, positioned as previously (and with a slightly firmer pressure) tap twice on each of the five points. Start with the rib directly below the armpit, move straight down to the last rib. Repeat in the same direction.

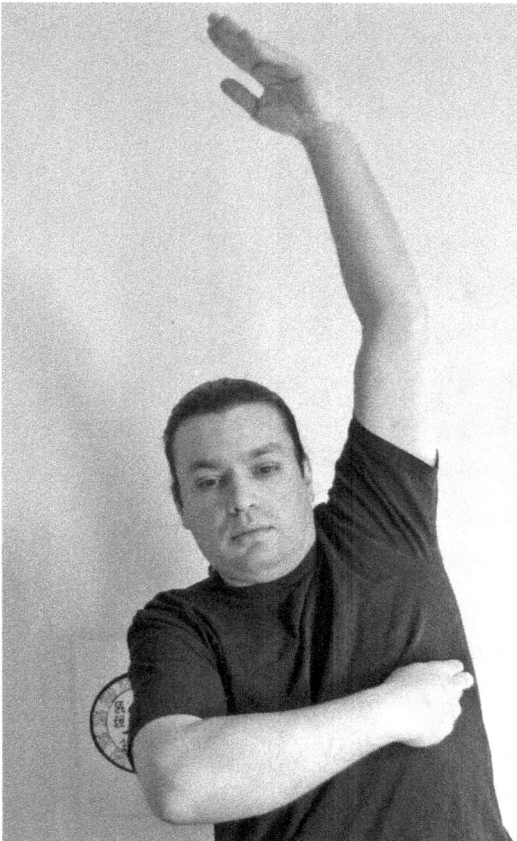

20. Saru Eleshar

Do the same procedure as in No. 19 on the right side, using the left hand.

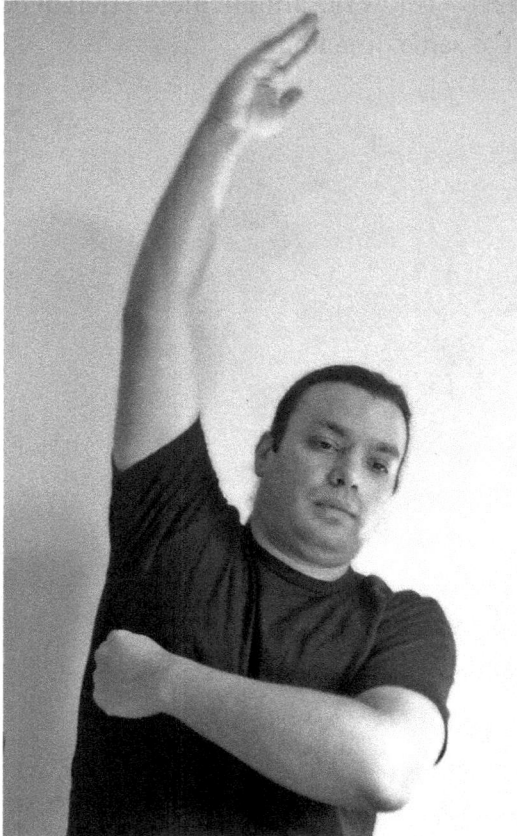

21. Nasu Anagu

The Nasu Anagu requires the same seated and hand postures as the previous postures. With the two fingers of each hand, tap the crown twice, the hands being 1.5" apart. Keeping the distance between the fingers, next tap the inner points of the eyebrows, then (the same distance apart) tap the top lip. Next tap the chin as illustrated on page 44. Each hand taps 4 points, twice each.

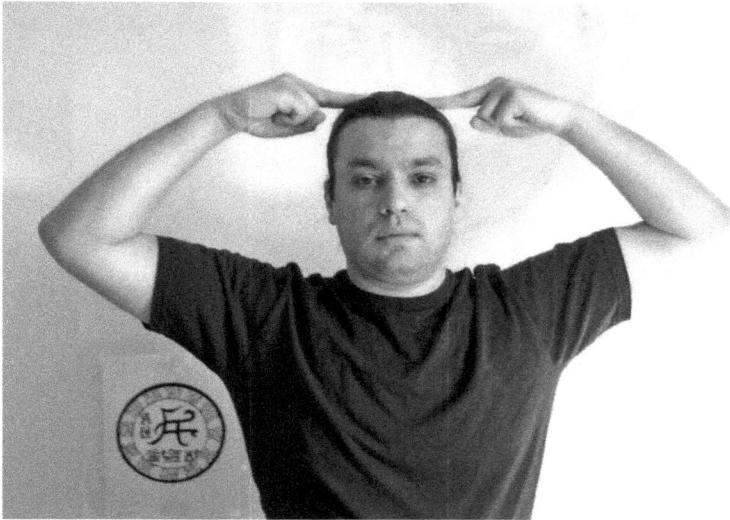

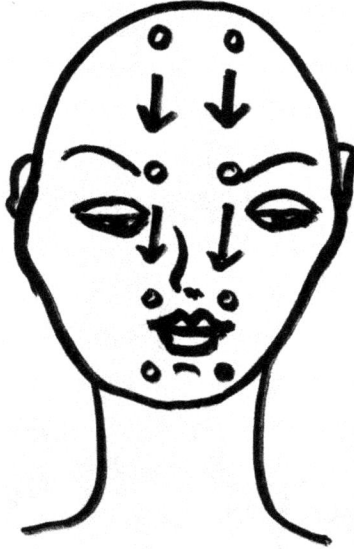

Nasu Anagu

Repeat for the duration of the sound elixir. The top
points are located on the crown.

22. Kaarsh-haras

Maintain the same postures as in No. 21. Using both hands, resting the middle finger on the top of the index finger, lightly tap twice the three points beneath the eyebrows on the brow bone — use *only* these fingers. Start above the tear duct and tap three points towards the ear as illustrated on page 46.

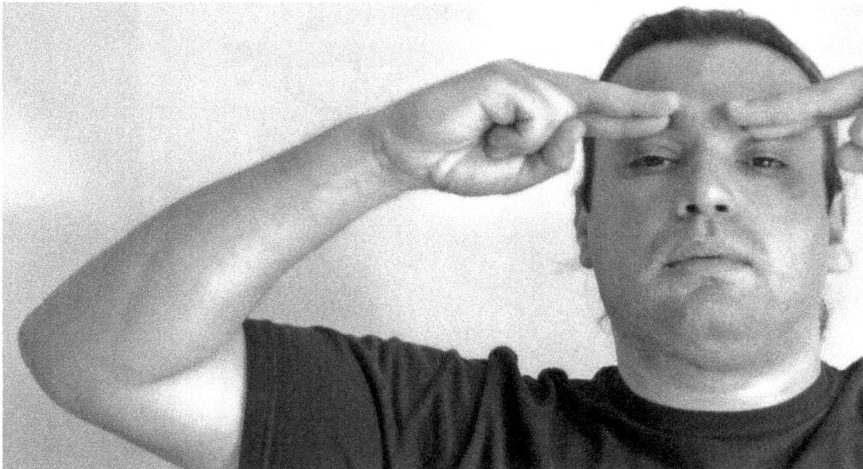

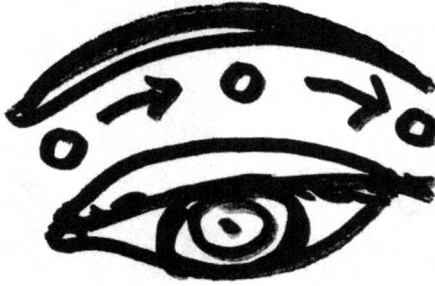

Kaarsh-haras

Start at the inner corner of the eye, under the brow,
repeat for the duration of the sound elixir.

23. Nistu Arana

Using the two index fingers tap twice the points under the chin (two points on each side) while the head is tilted back in a comfortable position. See the illustration, page 48: tap first the points located under the chin and then the points located 1" further outward and towards the ears.

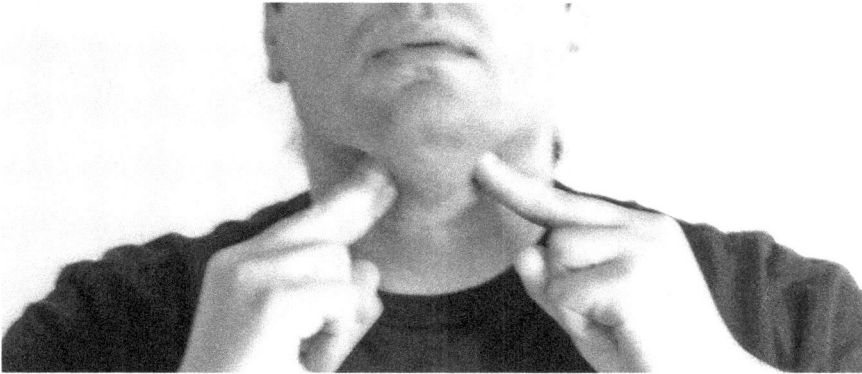

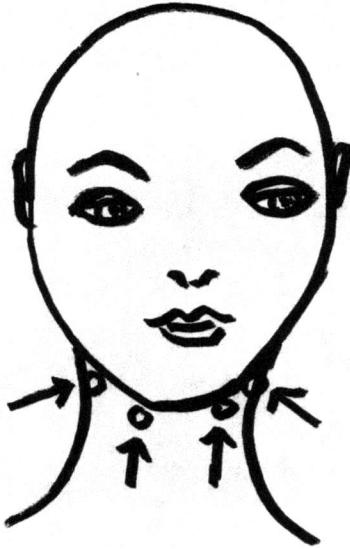

Nistu Arana

Repeat for the duration of the sound elixir.

24. Kivistu Branesh

With both hands, two fingers each, tap the chest bone (sternum) to the beat of the 24th elixir of the Mystical Kingdoms.

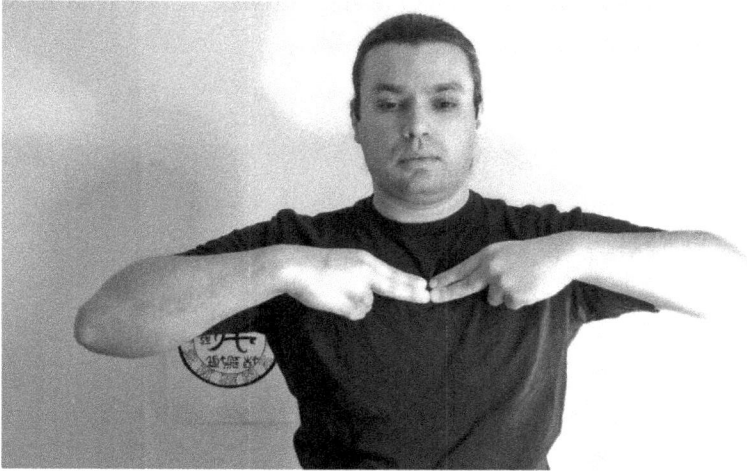

THE PRESSURE POSTURES – KUHULU-SATVI

25. Agnanut-havi

Lying comfortably on your mat with your arms crossed over your chest (left arm over right), use your thumbs to push with mild but steady pressure under the lowest point of your cheekbones. The right hand is pushing under the left cheekbone and vice versa. Maintain the pressure throughout the elixir.

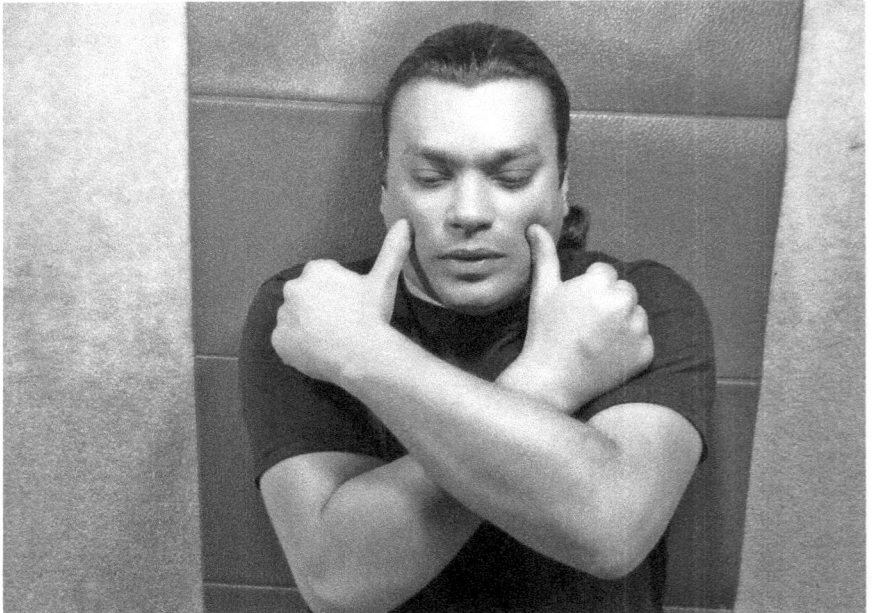

26. Bru-ak-nespahu

Lying comfortably, place your palms together and push with gentle pressure right behind and under your chin. With the tip of your tongue, push into the palate in the roof of your mouth. Maintain for the duration of the 26th elixir.

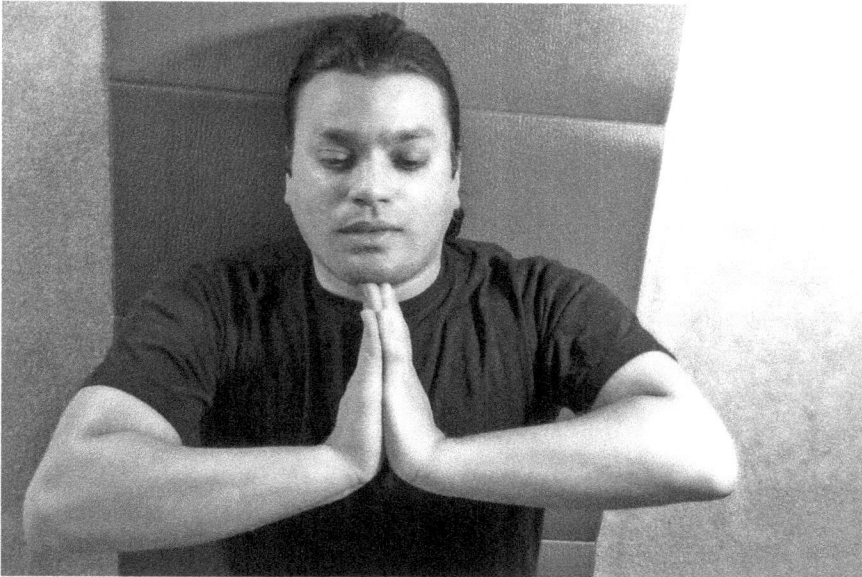

The Names of the 144 Gates

The Names of the Gates

Posture 1 – Ignati Rururet
1. Tranik-bilestra
2. Bruhat-bilshpavek
3. Uchnat-subarut

Posture 2 – Bligavesh
1. Misba-erekvit
2. Nisva-lu-uklat
3. Bri-es-varabit

Posture 3 – Bligavesh Iglat
1. Nik-his-astrava
2. Useta-manish
3. Helevis-asklata

Posture 4 – Bligavesh Uret
1. Vrihet-minavich
2. Vilevit-aleskla
3. Blinanut-prehut

Posture 5 – Nisavi Vishnatet
1. Arat-manavis
2. Arsk-usklata
3. Bravit-alesva

Posture 6 – Harasvu Isabi
1. Arisk-haratu
2. Urek-pilisba
3. Vravik-aresta

Posture 7 – Kunimani

1. Manich-bluhabat
2. Vrabis-estrava
3. Vrihet-alastar

Posture 8 – Ra-vanavish

1. Archpa-nunaves
2. Irek-blavabut
3. Nusaret-parabach

Posture 9 – Siti-vanavish

1. Nasarat-estava
2. Mishet-pluhabat
3. Naska-bilesta

Posture 10 – Rutga-vanavish

1. Arknit-ruspahur
2. Vli-eret-parabu
3. Misheta-arakskar

Posture 11 – Knanani-usubetvi

1. Sunavis-iresta
2. Bruharabit-mines
3. Rutska-vilivesbi

Posture 12 – Kasabi-usubetvi

1. Ararut-nictrava
2. Stu-uraves-vravi
3. Iriksava-mananus

Posture 13 – Kanatchi-esanum

1. Bluha-astravar
2. Rustamit-ananach
3. Suchmanet-uvar

4. Rutselvravi-arestar
5. Kri-es-ublafski
6. Pi-het-uru-seresasta

Posture 14 – Kushana-paarsi

1. Knuvrabar-skulavat
2. Virsta-bravabur
3. Arat-birevachspi
4. Rustel-mananech
5. Belhastru-krivesbi
6. Plihestratar-manuvish
7. Kenanut-esetar
8. Rutsalvanu-esevi
9. Plihar-minanes
10. Karsatur-ersklahut
11. Vri-erestravar
12. Virsbanut-eselvi
13. Rutbla-us-aresta
14. Arknesbra-ur
15. Urutna-bli-es
16. Iseter-milshpravi
17. Usuterak-nanaspu
18. Blives-aruspreha

Posture 15 – Nechsu-varish

1. Araktu-arskvranut
2. Rutselvrenot-raksparva
3. Virebat-raksprahur
4. Mishelva-urekspi
5. Akrat-unet-vravi
6. Blivebach-rutsabi
7. Miserut-alakstar

8. Pruhabit-urespi
9. Vriharanut-esetu
10. Alakbrihespar
11. Vru-unut-veresbi
12. Kaarnish-uvra
13. Prihet-alastar
14. Mishelvi-ukles
15. Stuvech-minesut

Posture 16 – Aasabi Plishet

1. Kersetu-manunes
2. Ristablu-vrihet
3. Stuvech-masarut
4. Mishtavu-ubeskvi
5. Prisetur-bliveset
6. Retspar-aresva
7. Nuchsate-plavish
8. Aruk-nastavi
9. Karuch-nesebit
10. Trevit-plavech-hustra
11. Arut-mines-aruspava
12. Tru-ha-nesvit
13. Ski-uhuranet
14. Pli-espravit

Posture 17 - Kanachvu

1. Ukrunasetuvi
2. Brihesplavit-urunes
3. Archba-spelevech
4. Virinat-arasketvavi
5. Blivabit-aravichvravi
6. Resetmanut-vrabit

If you want to win RFP business, you need to know how to write a winning proposal

There is more potential today—probably more than ever before—to increase business and achieve success by responding to Requests For Proposals (RFPs).

As they have for decades now, both government agencies and businesses rely increasingly on outsourcing to implement and complete projects. Whether it's a federal office looking for construction contractors to expand a facility, a state health agency looking for managed care organizations to run their Medicaid operations, or a local tech company looking to put in place a new computer network, organizations are increasingly turning to outside consultants and experts to get a job done.

How do they find those experts? The RFP.

RFPs are a doorway to contracts and opportunities. Literally billions of dollars are spent every year through RFPs, representing not just new income but new business for your company. The key is convincing the RFP issuer that you're the best choice to do the work for them.

And the way to do that is with a strong proposal that makes *you* the winner.

What makes a proposal successful? *Write the Winning Proposal* provides you proposal crafting tips and insights that have won over $8.1 billion in business for one writer's clients—tips that apply to any industry and to any proposal, small or large, and insights that can help you win contracts and grow your business.

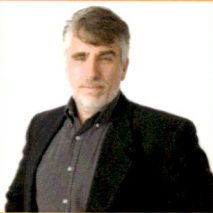

Patrick Dorsey is a writer and author with twenty-five years of experience leading winning technical and business communications projects in industries from aerospace to telecommunications to health care. He is the owner of St. Louis-based *Mightier Than The Sword Consulting,* where he creates successes helping people and businesses tell their stories.

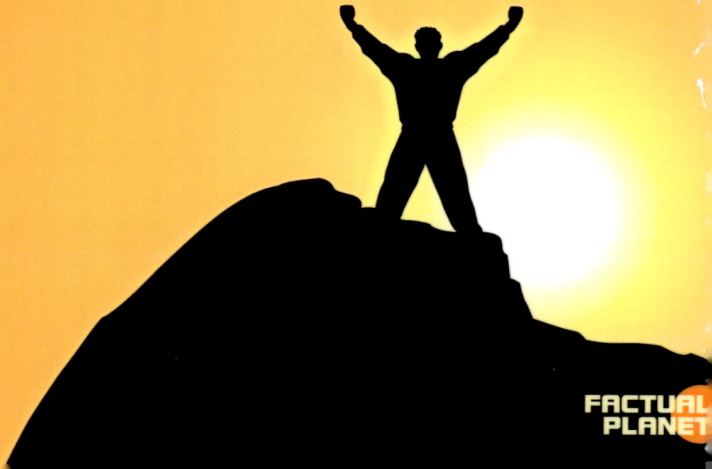

FACTUAL PLANET

7. Pelshpretahat
8. Isetusklavetvi
9. Iktra-balavushpi
10. Minach-bravabit
11. Erestrananur
12. Virechbravisbrahut

Posture 18 – Nasaar Isalvu
1. Nachsavu-uvesvi
2. Esetrar-manavis
3. Trihur-aranesbi
4. Sti-ablach-selvenus
5. Irkla-manavish
6. Rasba-useklet
7. Stri-ar-nananus
8. Krihastar-bravablut
9. Estre-miravech
10. Mesenusblavi-uset

Posture 19 – Saru Bishar
1. Astra-blavahur
2. Kretvi-mananur
3. Kruhas-estana
4. Bri-ihavestavar
5. Ninech-prihatur

Posture 20 – Saru Eleshar
1. Eresat-bravanesvi
2. Esekla-pravut
3. Vires-pravahur
4. Isetrach-trihabach
5. Arut-peleshavit

Posture 21 – Nasu Anagu

1. Nanusach-bravesti
2. Plihes-astava
3. Karanesvi-herspava
4. Niserach-uhabelesta
5. Bliset-arasta
6. Krihanach-spivarat
7. Mishtel-arasut
8. Esta-balishprava

Posture 22 – Kaarsh-haras

1. Niskavit-herastu
2. Kurastar-miserut
3. Nunech-aravesti
4. Mishata-nanusat
5. Klines-ersprahusvi
6. Si-utrer-nananesvi

Posture 23 – Nistu Arana

1. Kiretet-araskla
2. Bi-es-arastava
3. Urunur-kretplavi
4. Virenet-alsklar-manavish

Posture 24 – Kivistu Branesh

1. Kusuterenut-prava

Posture 25 – Aganut-havi

1. Biret-arasulesklar
2. Vri-uhurabet

Posture 26 – Bru-ak-nespahu

1. Misenat-kruhulesbi
2. Subavet-eklelchvi

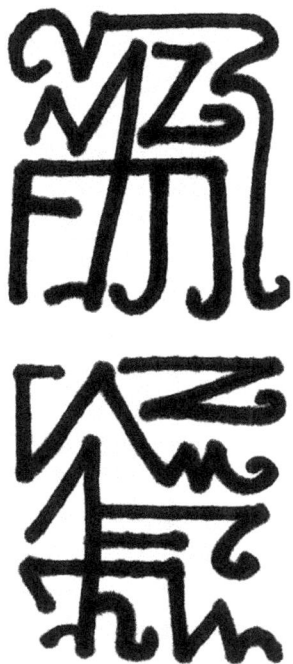

Understanding the
Abundance Principles

Principles: An Introduction

Comprehension and perception have always been the means of silencing our fears; fears of non-survival, of a depression or lack.

Instead of succumbing to the fears of the masses and becoming subject to manipulation by those who stand to gain from economic chaos, let us stand in mastery. Awareness of the principles that form the foundation of an abundant and prosperous life will help us achieve this.

Let us not lend strength to dire predictions of economic collapse. We are the creators of our own destinies. A re-vamping of our lives away from the debt-ridden sham that our economy has become is inevitable. We can weather the storm and survive.

The 144 Gates of Abundance

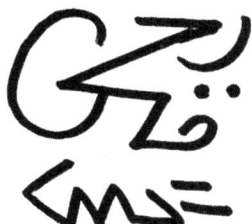

1. Necheratsatve

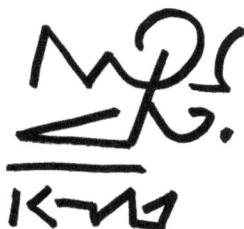

2. Mishinunask

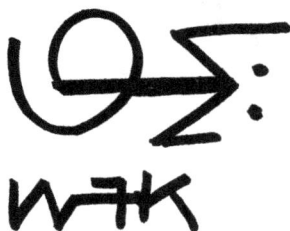

3. Sivibaratparve

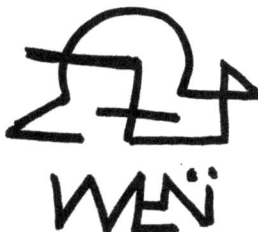

4. Neskavabrut

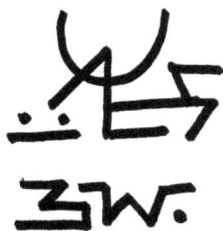

5. Kiha-usavava

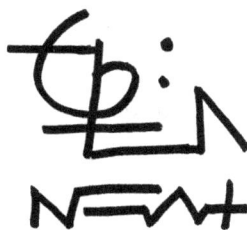

6. Blispa-ura

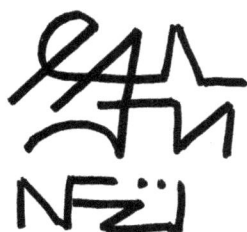

7. Kirina-ubelespetve

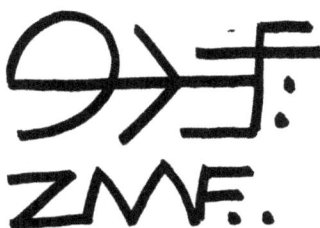

8. Nusarabi-eklavi

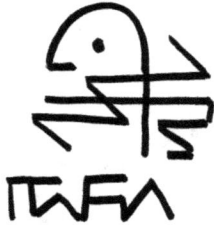

9. Usbakararu

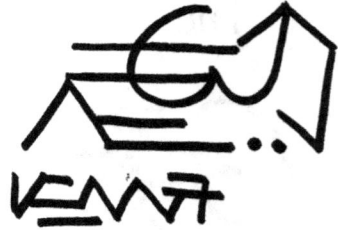

10. Utremishelvi

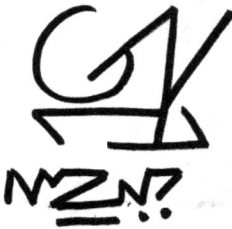

11. Archnat-husvavi

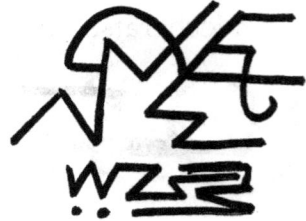

12. Truhenemenemi

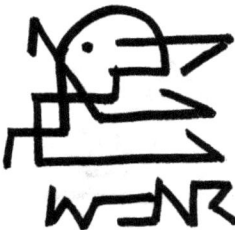

13. Sihubelvi-uvre

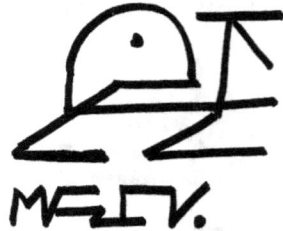

14. Kaarach-natvavesbi

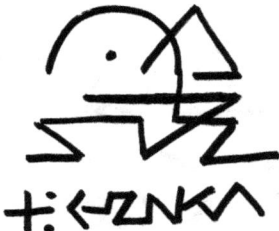

15. Sihuves-eklavi

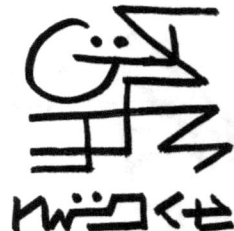

16. Nese-usalvavesbi

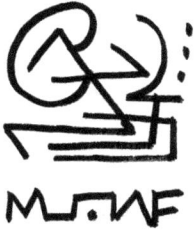

17. Iset-uhalesba

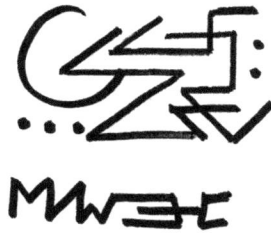

18. Achnaar-mishelvi

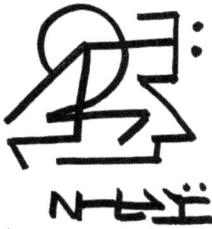

19. Kurastaar-birat

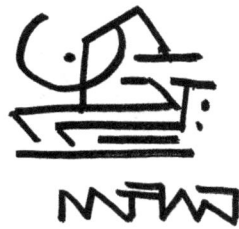

20. Utrenit-alsavi

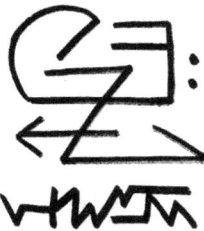

21. Bitru-echnaru

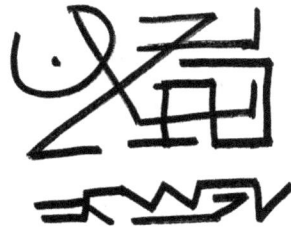

22. Kurstebitburet

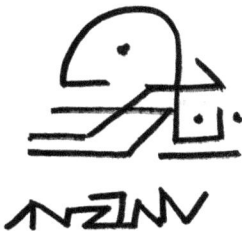

23. Kalahachbavrit

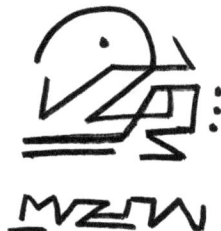

24. Nisalhuraspe

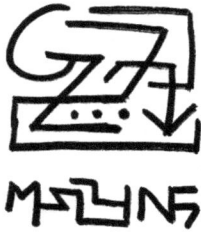

25. Pihurskalvavi

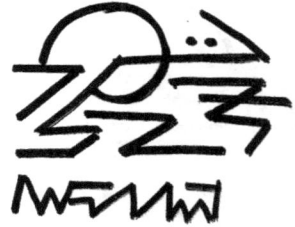

26. Ketrech-mishava

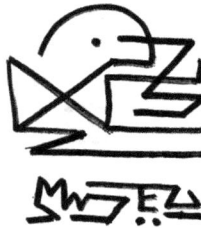

27. Ke-uhastar-esklavi

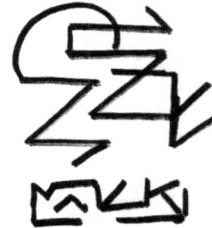

28. Sutulehunas

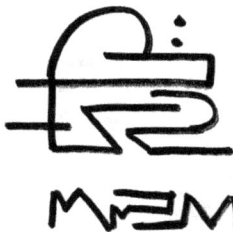

29. Verutbavelesvi

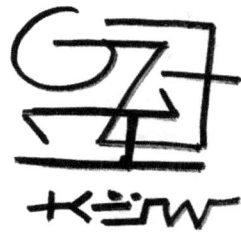

30. Karitmishba-el

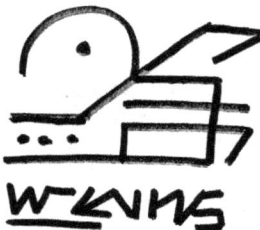

31. Otrunatskalva

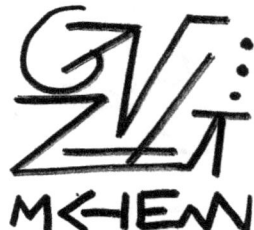

32. Ruchtavipa-hunat

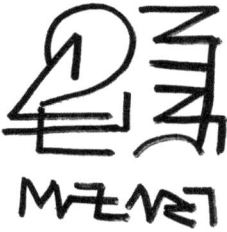

33. Kirasat-esalvi

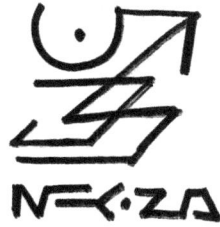

34. Sutelniserat

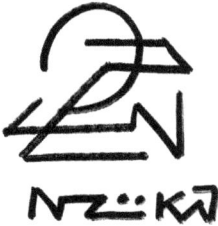

35. Kirabrutuhel

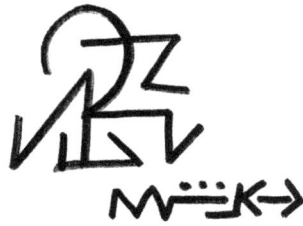

36. Nisabilevechvi

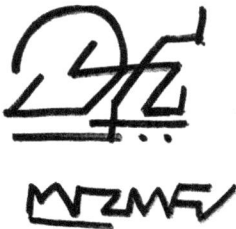

37. Arstapla-uhat

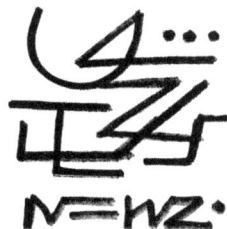

38. Vrusekba-esetu

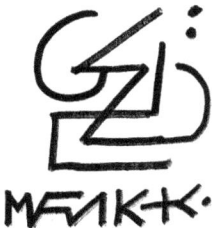

39. Trinimire-u-anat

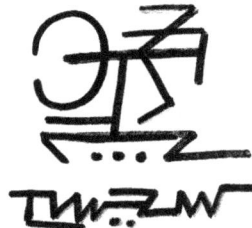

40. Keserut-aresta

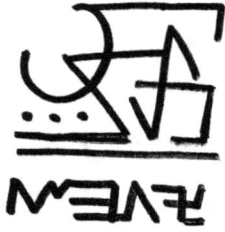

41. Vrutrubarus-esta

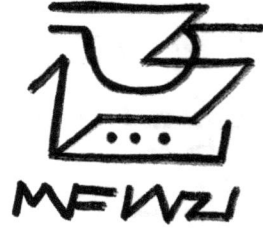

42. Kaarch-urasbi

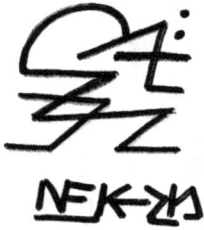

43. Sihasklava

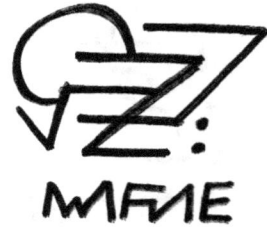

44. Erkba-usenetvi

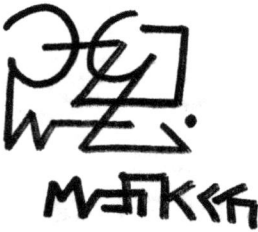

45. Kira-sivelvru

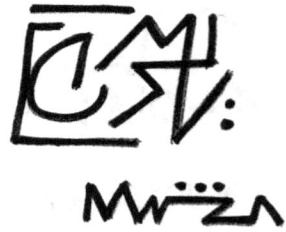

46. Isel-iselka-uha

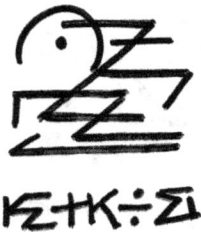

47. Nusbararut-uklave

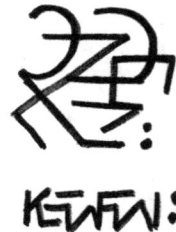

48. Kuritmistu-vibrat

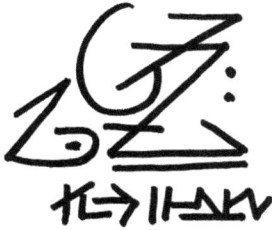

49. Arathurspaklavit

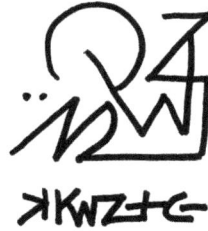

50. Arutprevitprahur

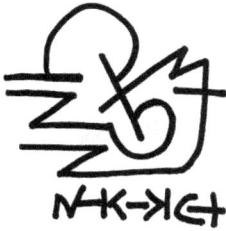

51. Kununisarsta

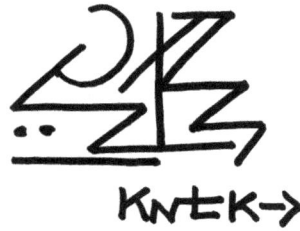

52. Virenimespahur

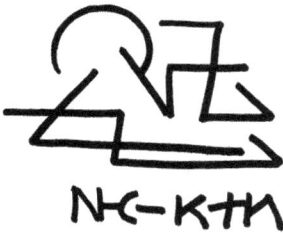

53. Archarnot

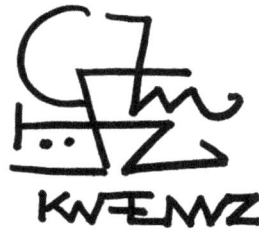

54. Vilshpaver

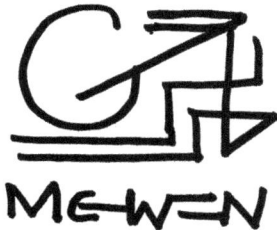

55. Useta-minaruch

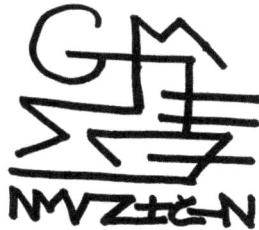

56. Harasut-ekleva

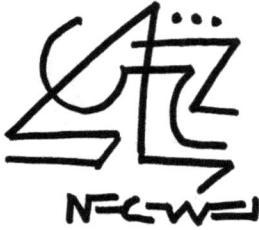

57. Urchbarut-harestu

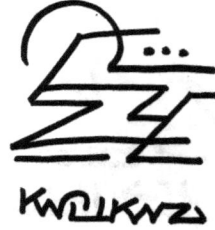

58. Nesaretvibarish

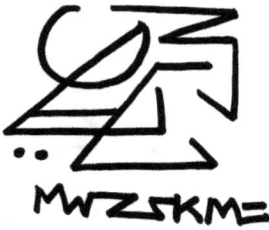

59. Usutu-hesklave

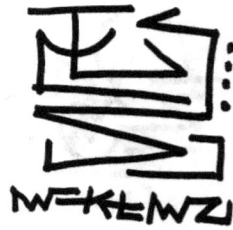

60. Erklevibrasiva-el

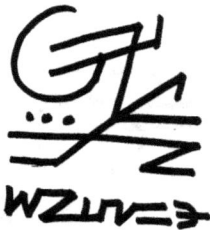

61. Arknipribasuvael

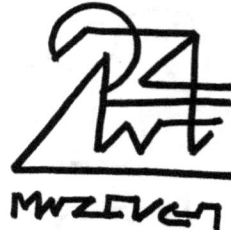

62. Esete-mishavi

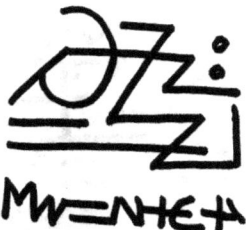

63. Nisitrananuspavel

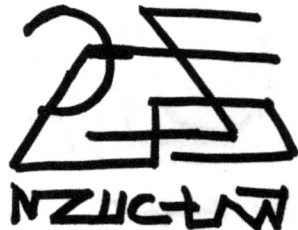

64. Uklevisa-usba-el

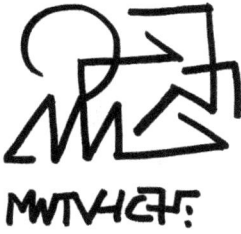

65. Uhuvrasut-ekenechvi-vavru

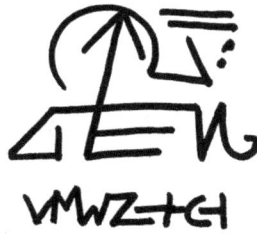

66. Asabitvaret

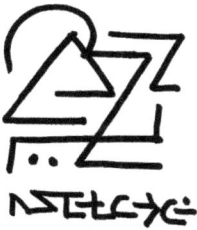

67. Kuhele-ustrava

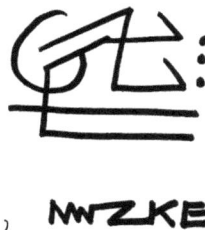

68. Kese-usalava

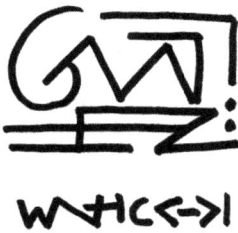

69. Husalnanetkleva

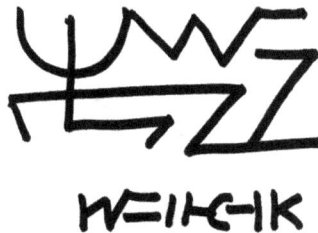

70. Ruchperpranavishper

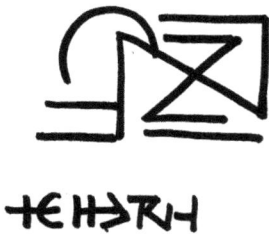

71. Nuselvevarabi

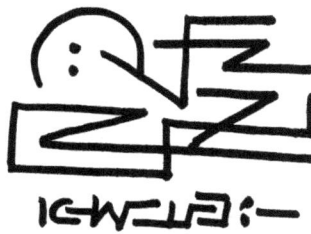

72. Aktrahanesetu

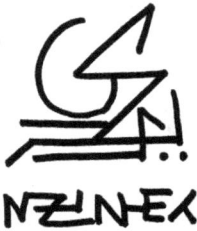

73. Ruchtrerig-ashva

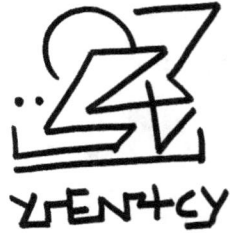

74. Oselena-skavir

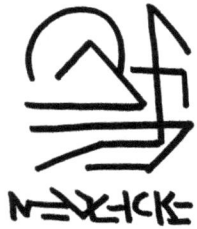

75. Utrekverbitvranu

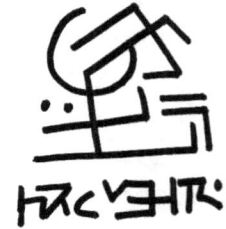

76. Kirsprahu

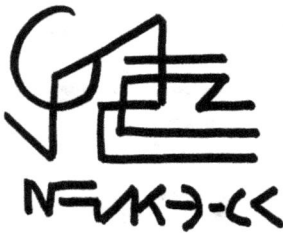

77. Sitklevrenavu

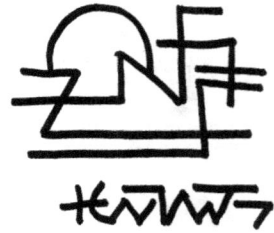

78. Uskeleperenu

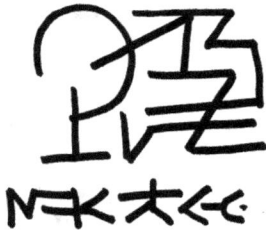

79. Aktrabar-rutvavi

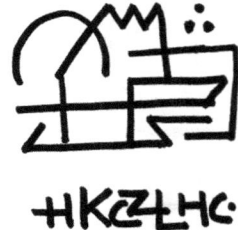

80. Petribarprevu

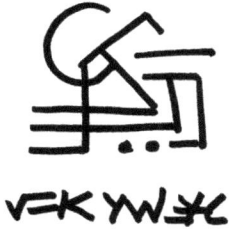

81. Arekstavar-aresni

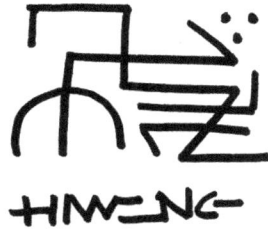

82. Husetminur-haresbi

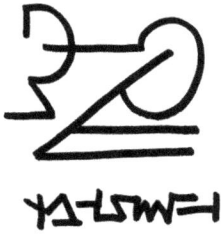

83. Eklevibretsalvavu

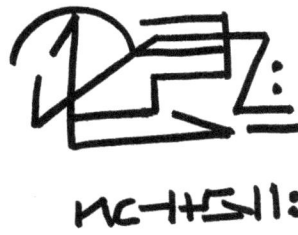

84. Archpa-minurparvet

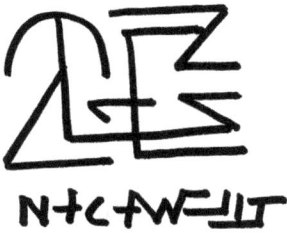

85. Lispera-unesvi

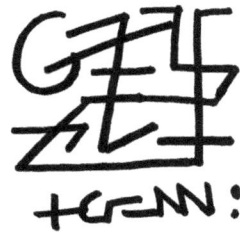

86. Rikpertresubar

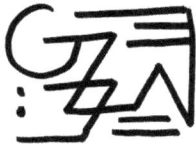

87. Iselvri-isevechvi

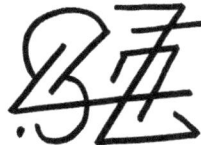

88. Niset-arusprehit

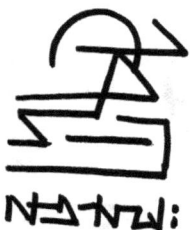

89. Kiranut-useltra

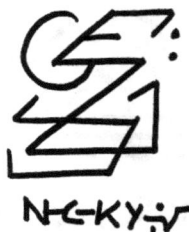

90. Viselvu-nisbaret

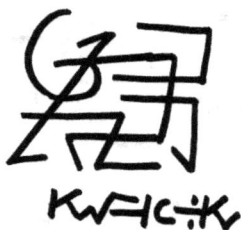

91. Kelhe-etrevibareru

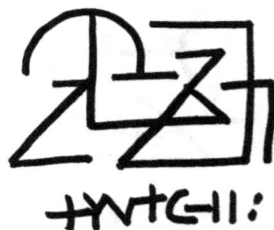

92. Nachpa-blavushvi

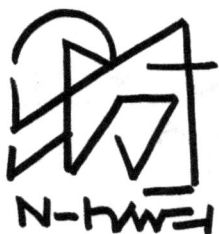

93. Arusparva-kererut

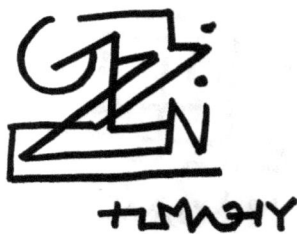

94. Haris-esklavu

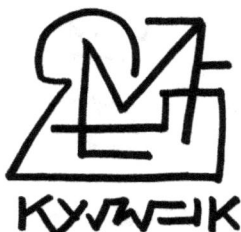

95. Suthit-arsevrunu

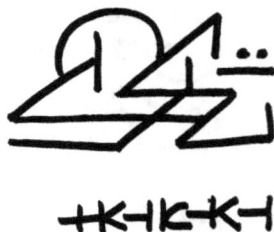

96. Viblik-aretvrenut

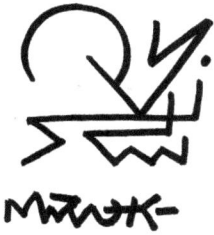

97. Sutvaa-arsekla

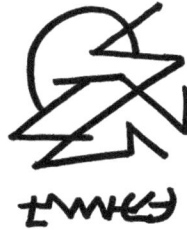

98. Etsilbihar-nursta

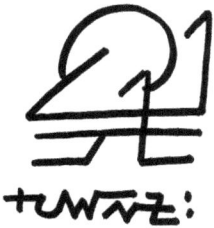

99. Karuchpaher-uset

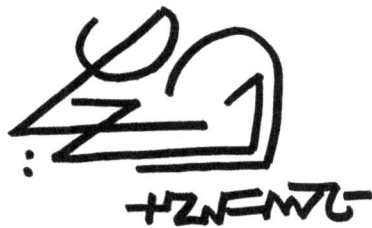

100. Klivabrahutspanu

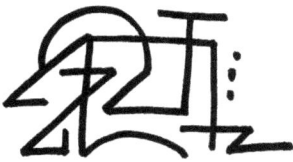

101. Esetepirahet

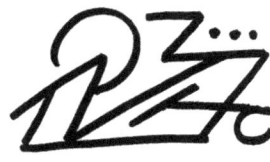

102. Viripamichba-er

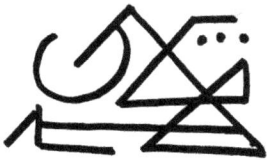

103. Kassabi-unaset

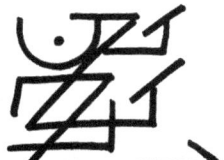

104. Vibri-unar-sklava

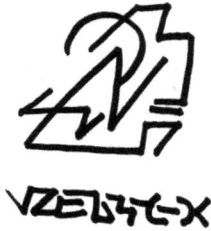

105. Situmisanesparhu

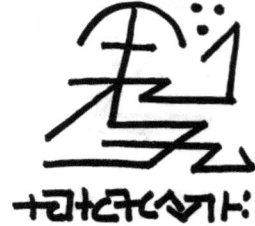

106. Viblesaraskranit

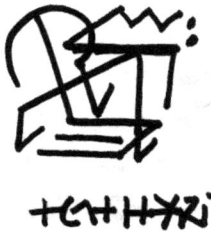

107. Usatblanich-serut

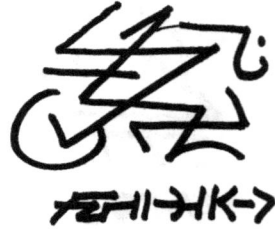

108. Arska-ekletvibrat

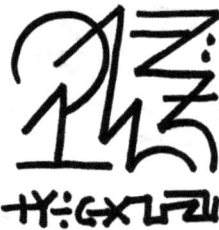

109. Iseta-nachsparut

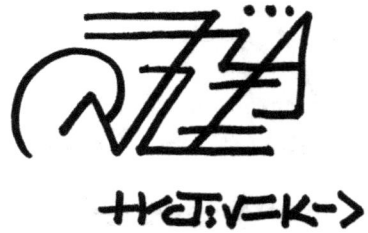

110. Ukluvris-aranasut

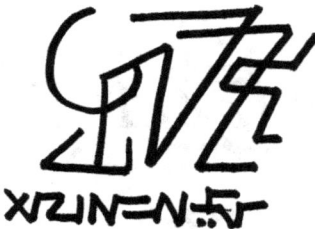

111. Eseteprahut-arsta

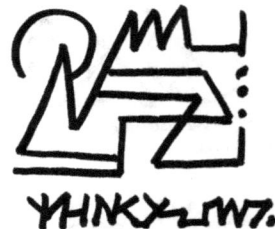

112. Vilinisperut-ukle

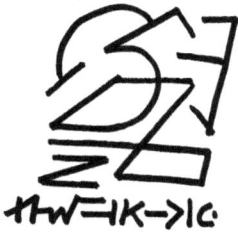

113. Kaalanat-uset

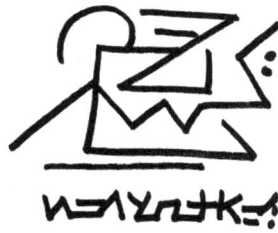

114. Etre-minis-verspa

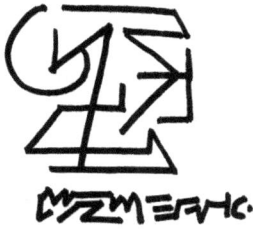

115. Kuhut-alerklesbi

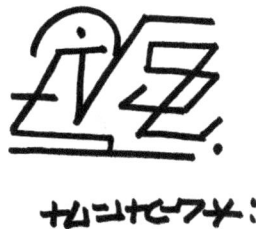

116. Archpa-isetnut

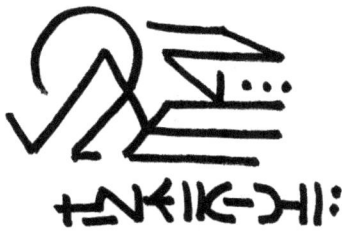

117. Hutre-viliset

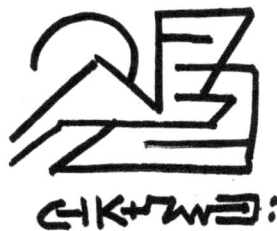

118. Eskle-minirus

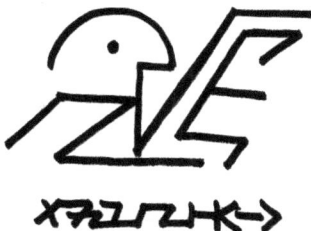

119. Urutrakve-irespa

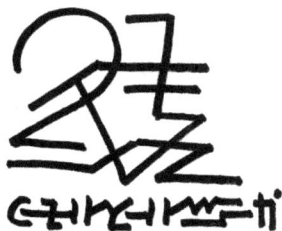

120. Uharanatve-vilevis

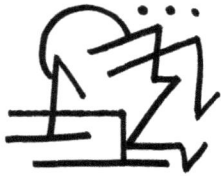

121. Usanandabi

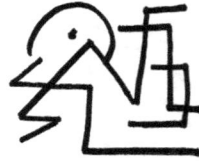

122. Ekselvrivar

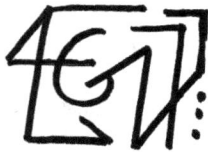

123. Aknaspraruspleha

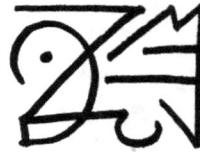

124. Utunasvevrubahar

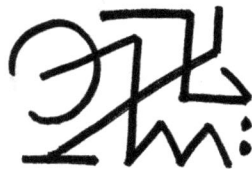

125. Archnitvrevasusklar

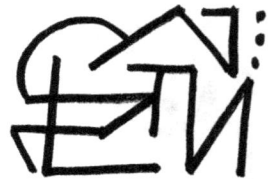

126. Perenut-vrehasversklu

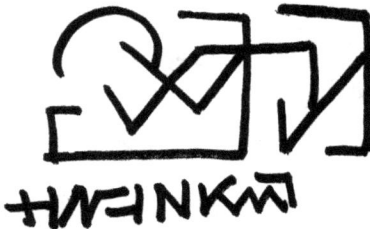

127. Kelsat-plahuranes

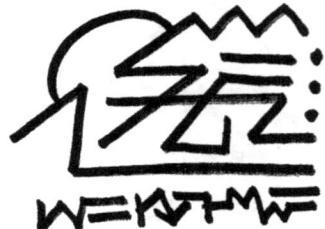

128. Vivarek-minestra

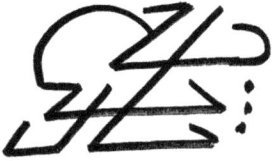

129. Usaba-vibelestu

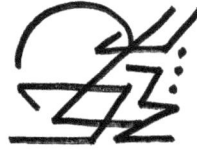

130. Asanahuspeva

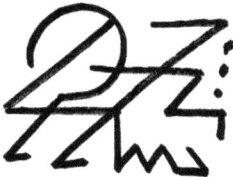

131. Kaarsabitekla

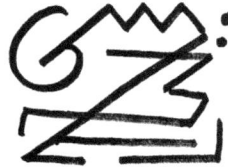

132. Vrubelelchnu-avi

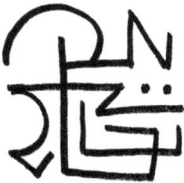

133. Velspa-urektrana

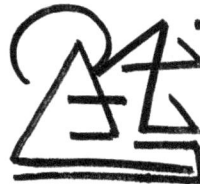

134. Mishpaplihenut

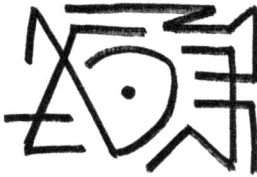

135. Ukle-viberestrevanu

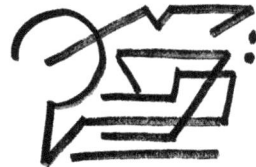

136. Asanahu

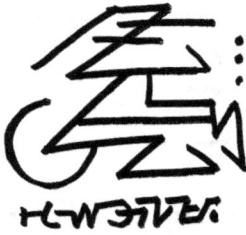

137. Plevi-avi

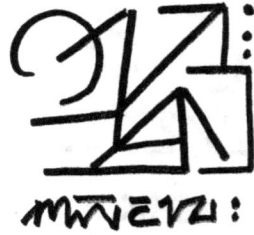

138. Haarechnesba-aleskla

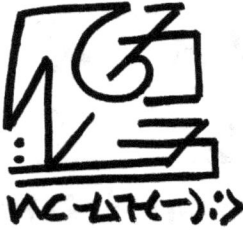

139. Sitinatvi-perere

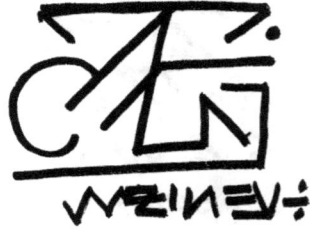

140. Iktranu-speklu-aha

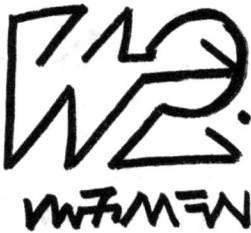

141. Avanet-hilsba

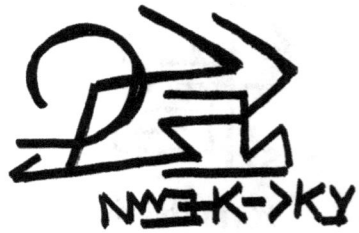

142. Usekparuspa-ekleva

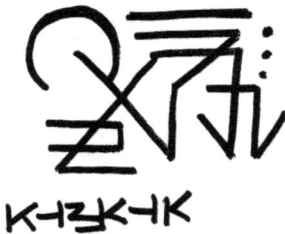

143. Visarat-minechvires

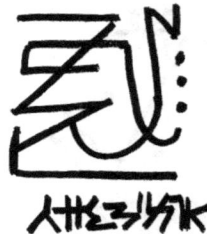

144. Kivaranut-preha

The 144 Principles of Abundance

1. Acknowledgement of the source of all abundance as ourselves giving to ourselves increases the flow.
2. The flow of abundance is an illusion. We have always had access to all abundance.
3. Let our daily mantra be "I am abundance."
4. To consider the recipient's worth when giving is to close the sluices of our supply, for to deny another's worth is to deny ourselves.
5. To think of money as a base currency is to forget that all that exists is the One Life.
6. The illusion of relationship is a game for the sake of delight. Money is a man-made game within a game and should also be for delight.
7. Abundance is living within your means with grace. It has nothing to do with how much you have or earn.
8. The viewpoint that money must be earned reduces the possibility that it can come from other sources.
9. Treating ourselves with abundant care and nurturing is the first step to an abundant life.
10. The true currency of an abundant life is elegance combined with grace born of self-respect and is available to all.
11. Treat money with respect. It is the thread that weaves together the tapestry of human societies.
12. Send a blessing with the money you spend, that it may bless the fisherman and statesman alike.
13. Money is the man-made lifeblood of society. It circulates, bringing back to you that which you send out with it.
14. When we see our monetary resources as our security, we deny that our being is our sustenance.

15. When money becomes the measuring stick of our achievements, our desire for wealth becomes an obsession.

16. To desire to live abundantly is as natural as the fish desiring the ocean. Money is only a small part of abundance.

17. Be lavish with yourself with those things that bring you joy. Awareness helps us find joy in simple pleasures.

18. To regret the loss of resources is to deny that we are the creators of our lives and can create as much abundance again.

19. Some feel guilt at having too much and others at having too little. Guilt clogs the arteries of supply.

20. Some acquire to live, others live to acquire. In both instances acquisition has become a need rather than a joy.

21. As the One Life, we are all things; there is nothing to become. When we strive for more, we perpetuate impoverishment.

22. Vigorously uproot belief systems that indoctrinate with perceived status symbols and fabricated needs.

23. The weight of comparisons will impede us as we dance with the abundance of life.

24. Comparisons will either make us feel poor because we have less or guilty because we think we have more. Each one has manifested their life in divine perfection. Let us honor this.

25. In seeing the poverty of another we are observing an impoverished part of ourselves. Fix within what is imperfect without.

26. When we bargain we bar ourselves from gain. The law of compensation decrees that life too will then short-change us.

27. Spend only what you have so that you do not become the slave of dysfunctional needs.

28. Budgets block the torrential flow of abundance. Plan, but hold lightly to your plans and expect abundant surprises.

29. As you wish for abundance, ask for the world if that is what you want. If your desire is not met, no matter – it was not a need but a preference.
30. Stagnation of resources comes from ruts. Let the adventure of life unfold anew in your life daily.
31. If you desire flow to come to your life, do not hoard. Donate that which you do not use and throw away clutter.
32. See yourself as a steward of your possessions. Treat them with respect and repair rather than replace them whenever practical.
33. Those who take in greed deplete not only themselves but others as well.
34. Taking resources for granted depletes them. All things dwindle in the face of ingratitude.
35. When we approach anything with the question of "What is the most I can get?" scarcity arises. Let us approach food with appreciation rather than a need for nutrition.
36. When we listen to our inner rhythms our lives become fertile. Barrenness arises when we do not listen to the song of our heart.
37. Loss of possessions is viewed by some as equivalent to loss of life. It is often the catalyst to deeper living and vitality.
38. A life of simplicity is not more enlightened than a life of complexity. It just removes the temptation of having our possessions possess us.
39. Find the true pleasures of life. Man, having lost touch with what brings him joy, substitutes the veneer of purchased sophistication.
40. Live life as a work of art. Let an attitude of graceful creativity enliven your financial affairs.

41. Paint life with a large brushstroke, but do not neglect the details. So too in financial affairs where small leakages can drain the reservoir of resources.

42. In times of scarcity know it to be a temporary re-grouping that will reveal what really matters.

43. When resources are scarce, let innovation blossom. This in itself can be a form of creativity shared with others.

44. Adversity can teach us and our family more than many years of prosperity only if we enthusiastically pick up the gauntlet.

45. Life cannot take away without compensating us. A hole cannot be made in the ocean. Watch for new areas of abundance.

46. It is through asking for what we want, while appreciating what we have, that we live the most powerful law of abundance.

47. Each family member has a psychological poverty consciousness trigger. The housewife may need a supply of canned food to feel abundant. As far as possible, honor these triggers for your family.

48. We are in a society that lures us into debt as a way of life. Resist this insanity as much as possible. Save first, then buy. Your greatest asset is freedom.

49. Not only is debt a form of enslavement, but it creates the unwholesome situation where we do not own the food we eat or the clothes we wear – the bank does.

50. How do we reduce a burden of debt? Get professional assistance and as in any long journey, do it one step at a time.

51. All addictions are the result of self-abandonment. The addiction of spending is no different. Balanced spending comes from balanced living.

52. The financial dynamics of a family unit indicate its flow of power. Where the assets and monetary control is lodged, there too is the power.

53. Money is crystallized power and the same laws apply. When it is hoarded, the universe conspires to take it away.

54. Life's fertility wanes when there's egocentricity. Spontaneous giving of the self creates an environment in which to flourish.

55. When life becomes consumed with duty, the heart feels deprived. Life becomes impoverished. No money can compensate for that.

56. Envision carefully what you wish to manifest. Return to it several times a day, adding more detail. See it as though it already exists.

57. Spend money as a proxy. As you give a dollar to a person in need, give it by proxy through intention to all who are in need.

58. In treating money as crystallized power, with intention empower what you spend money on. Taxes create amenities that better society - envision that.

59. The monetary system uses counterfeit value, pretending paper money has value. It must evolve to a barter system and beyond.

60. The ultimate goal of the evolution of the monetary system is that we offer goods or services for what they are intrinsically worth to us in trade – a voluntary trade system.

61. The evolution into a barter and voluntary trade system must begin with us – even if it is just one step at a time.

62. The communities of the future will function from a trust system where all put their products and services to use and take what they need.

63. Frugality has nothing to do with how much we spend, but in how impeccably we refuse to squander energy through playing dysfunctional games with others and through resisting life.
64. When we labor with joy and excellence, drudgery to earn a living turns to a labor of love and creativity.
65. Send blessings with your work that the fruits of your labor may have increased value and leave the cosmos in your debt.
66. A production line can become a mantra when our attitude is one of voluntary service to all life.
67. Acknowledge with gratitude those who serve you and life will support you.
68. In life's dealings, give the most you can and not the least. Otherwise you leave yourself in life's debt.
69. Surround yourself with those who, like you, seek to give the most possible so that you are supported by winners.
70. Shun those who seek the most they can get, that you may not be encumbered by parasitic vines.
71. There are those who seek to diminish your resources and achievements and those who try and profit from them. Neither believes they can achieve through their own efforts.
72. Enabling others to view you as their line of credit is to promote disempowerment and a misplaced sense of entitlement.
73. If you give to another, consider the extent of his need. He may need a skill, or to be put in touch with an agency or a month's rent. Next, consider your capacity to give.
74. Give that you may get. He who generously assists where he can, opens the sluices of cosmic supply.
75. Where families have been supported by large debt structures, a necessary economic re-adjustment is to be expected. Substance must replace such hollowness.

76. To the caterpillar in the cocoon, his metamorphosis seems catastrophic. The financial system likewise must transfigure.
77. Do not lend empowerment through attention to financial doomsday predictions. Prepare for the worst and expect the best.
78. Trust in the resilience and ingenuity of man and in one lending a helping hand to another to successfully navigate a global recession.
79. Let recovery from financial setbacks become a family affair that children may learn how to cheerfully and optimistically adjust to life's vicissitudes.
80. Life presents daily doors for you to knock on. Be alert to these multiple opportunities. Some may open and some may not, but knock!
81. Do not hang back from knocking on doors before you because you do not know whether you want to enter. Wonderful surprises may lie across that threshold.
82. Instead of spending energy on casting blame, winners spend it in accomplishing. This creates the opportunity for life to even the score by recompensing you.
83. Failure is not lack of success, it is being afraid to try.
84. To measure our success by possessions is to be enslaved by the false values of social conditioning.
85. Self-pity creates a downward spiral in our circumstances, since what we focus on increases.
86. Self-importance stemming from past accomplishments and pride of possessions blocks the manifestation of an even greater future.
87. Fluidity is the key factor of success in financially trying times. Consider temporary options and multiple jobs.

88. Time management is essential when demands increase. Use a structured and disciplined approach, leaving time for fun with loved ones.
89. The Earth groans under the weight of refuse from prepared food containers. Returning to whole foods is not only economical, but a return to conscious living.
90. Scientists have found we entrain the Earth and vice versa. When we cultivate fertile gardens, the Earth restores our fertile abundance.
91. By cutting ourselves off from nature we lose sight of sound values and become steeped in blind materialism.
92. Knowing the Earth to be our source of supply and our being to be our sustenance, we have established the foundations for prosperity.
93. Think of money as love. Give freely where you can and it will return freely.
94. Would you bargain with your love, giving only as little as you can? Then why would you bargain and withhold money?
95. To allow ourselves to pay the over-inflated prices masquerading as sophisticated trendiness is to support self-important exploitation of society.
96. By doing your work with a glad heart, as a service to life, you become a cause rather than an effect.
97. All successful achievers know that they write the script of the play of their lives. As they see themselves as abundant, so they become.
98. In taking time for deep meaningful living, like watching the dawn, we know our joy. Joy is the guidance system for our choices.

99. Living from the fully conscious life of wholesome values puts substance behind our endeavors. Soulless activity is hollow and cannot support abundance.

100. Do not let your work dictate the pace of your life. Dedicate time slots in which you respond to its demands. In this way it does not become the master and you the slave.

101. Neither abundance nor poverty exists within the Ocean of Life. When we know this, we are free.

102. To see poverty in another is to disacknowledge the cosmic compensation for any seeming loss.

103. Greed is born from seeing resources as limited, which in turn comes from living a life of boundaries.

104. It does not matter how many hours you work if there is creativity, passion and excellence being expressed; work has changed from duty to joyous life.

105. Create a home, not a house - a place in which reverence is given to the divinity of those who dwell in it.

106. Homemaking should be regarded as a form of worship through service.

107. Create in whatever measure you can, a work and living environment that expresses reverence for life as sacred.

108. Tolerance and respect for others does not mean you should allow disrespect of the sacred space in which you live and work.

109. There is no form of work more important than another when all is done as an offer of love upon the altar of life.

110. Many find bankruptcy unacceptable and immoral when huge amounts of money were spent to incur the debt in the first place.

111. To refuse to declare bankruptcy when extricating oneself from debt through other means is impossible, is like the moth refusing to leave the spider's web on 'moral grounds'.
112. When we learn our lessons, life does not repeat or prolong hardship. Life is an adventure of insight, not a punitive taskmaster.
113. Karmic repercussions for debt cannot exist, since there is no time and within the One Life debt is an illusion.
114. Guilt over incurred debt blocks future flow. Any beneficial change requires acceptance of the present.
115. Man microcosmically represents the debt Creation has accrued by using the resources of the Infinite's Embodiment after cosmic supply became scarce.
116. Abundance requires not only directed flow through generosity, but containment. Allowing waste and drainage amounts to trying to contain abundance in a sieve.
117. Those who flourish in hard financial times are those who find creative solutions, rather than focusing on the problems.
118. When financial systems fail us, looking for solutions within that failed system seldom works. Think outside the box.
119. Redefine abundance as having all you need and not needing all you have. Most mistakenly regard extravagant excess as abundance.
120. Your possessions are your stewardship. Repair them rather than discarding, that the garbage heaps on Earth may dwindle.
121. Help where you can, but do not feel guilt about having while others do not. Uniformity stifles a society's development.
122. Whatever you manifested before, your being is as capable of doing the same or better again. Live with hope and without regrets.

123. To create a new paradigm of living, simplify your life so that the life-enhancing aspects may reveal themselves.
124. The soul justifies its excesses and indulgences through self-pity. Uproot self-pity ruthlessly – it obscures truth.
125. Self-pity looks outside itself to be rescued. Self-responsibility finds a solution.
126. Simplifying life, like cooking with staples rather than pre-packaged food, requires more time but reduces waste and expenditure.
127. By reducing acquisition, appreciation is found for what we have. Always looking beyond the horizon leaves the surrounding landscape unappreciated.
128. Believe in the bounty of life and claim it as your own by living generously and avoiding hoarding.
129. Do not use money as a substitute for giving of yourself. It creates an imbalance of lack for you and others.
130. Principles of abundance are first learnt within the heart. When we give with joy, resources multiply.
131. When we allow others to take from us and pillage our lives, our time and our resources, we keep them from accomplishing on their own.
132. Massive industries and institutions are built to feed on the achievements and misfortunes of others. Surround yourself with those who believe in their own accomplishments.
133. Allowing those who unsuccessfully manage their own lives to manage part of yours, is as foolish as the patient trying to treat the physician.
134. Judge not a slow pace as more praiseworthy than a fast one. In timelessness the concept of pace does not exist.

135. Celebrate success but do not take it seriously. Neither success nor failure can be ours when there is only One Life expressing.

136. Success and abundance are the only constants in life. We either align ourselves with them through surrender and trust, or cut ourselves off from them through opposing life.

137. Contemplate with praise the abundance of the stars, the snowflakes, the field flowers. For what you focus on, you become.

138. We dwell in an ocean of abundance. We are limited only by our ability to recognize what is available.

139. Abundance is a bottomless pit when it is defined as increase. We live in elegant sufficiency when we gratefully recognize we have all we need.

140. Self-confidence assumes incorrectly that it must create what it needs. Humility recognizes the self as a conduit for eternal flow.

141. Many feel guilt because they have more, while others feel guilt because they have less. There will always be alternating areas within beingness where certain resources are more emphasized. Equalization produces mediocrity.

142. When certain resources are emphasized in an individual's life, others are de-emphasized. Discover with gratitude where your wealth lies.

143. When we neglect the feminine[7] within ourselves, our receptivity to abundance becomes inactive and life becomes barren.

144. When you receive and hoard, you have become the tomb of abundance. When you receive and give, you are the womb of abundant flow.

---

7 See the Goddess Archetypes in *Journey to the Heart of God.*

Other books by Almine

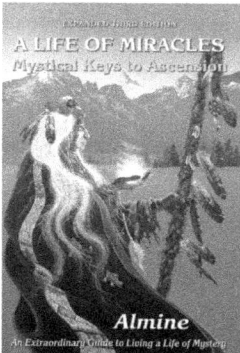

A Life of Miracles
Expanded Third Edition IncludesBonus Belvaspata
Section—Mystical Keys to Ascension
Almine's developing spiritual awareness and abilities from
her childhood in South Africa until she emerged as a powerful mystic, to devote her gifts in support of all humanity is
traced. Deeply inspiring and unique in its comparison of
man's relationship as the microcosm of the macrocosm.
Also available in Spanish.

Published: 2009, 304 pages, soft cover, 6 x 9, ISBN: 978-1-934070-25-3

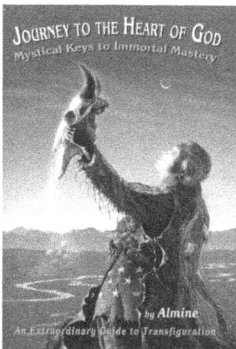

Journey to the Heart of God *Second Edition*
Mystical Keys to Immortal Mastery
Ground-breaking cosmology revealed for the first time, sheds
new light on previous bodies of information such as the
Torah, the I Ching and the Mayan Zolkien. The   explanation of man's relationship as the microcosm as set out in the
previous book *A Life of Miracles*, is expanded in a way never
before addressed by New Age authors, giving new meaning
and purpose to human life. Endorsed by an Astro-physicist
from Cambridge University and a former NASA scientist,
this book is foundational for readers at all levels of spiritual
growth.

Published: 2009, 296 pages, soft cover, 6 x 9, ISBN: 978-1-934070-26-0

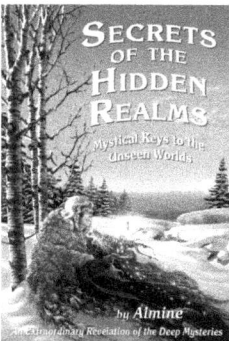

Secrets Of The Hidden Realms *Second Edition*
Mystical Keys to the Unseen Worlds
This remarkable book delves into mysteries few mystics have
ever revealed. It gives in detail: *The practical application of the
goddess mysteries • Secrets of the angelic realms • The maps,
alphabets, numerical systems of Lemuria, Atlantis, and the Inner
Earth • The Atlantean calender, accurate within 5 minutes • The
alphabet of the Akashic libraries. Secrets of the Hidden Realms*
is a truly amazing bridge across the chasm that has separated
humanity for eons from unseen realms.

Published: 2009, 412 pages, soft cover, 6 x 9, ISBN: 978-1-934070-27-7

Other books by Almine

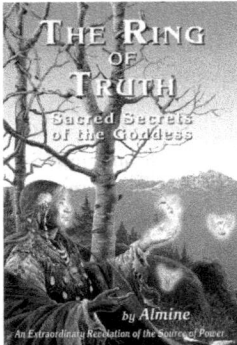

The Ring of Truth *Third Edition*
Sacred Secrets of the Goddess
As man slumbers in awareness, the nature of his reality has altered forever. As one of the most profound mystics of all time, Almine explains this dramatic shift in cosmic laws that is changing life on earth irrevocably. A powerful healing modality is presented to compensate for the changes in laws of energy, healers have traditionally relied upon. The new principles of beneficial white magic and the massive changes in spiritual warriorship are meticulously explained.

Published: 2009, 256 pages, soft cover, 6 x 9, ISBN: 978-1-934070-28-4

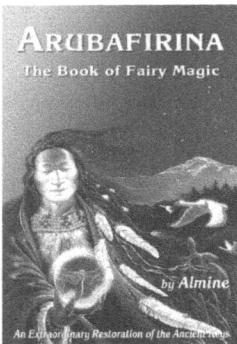

Arubafirina *Second Edition*
The Book of Fairy Magic
This book is most certainly a milestone in the history of mysticism throughout the ages. It is the product of a rare and unprecedented event in which Almine, acknowledged as the leading mystic of our time, was granted an exceptional privilege. For one week in November 2006 she was invited to enter the fairy realms and gather the priceless information for this book. The result is a tremendous treasure trove of knowledge and interdimensional color photos.

Published: 2009, 196 pages, soft cover, 6 x 9, ISBN: 978-1-934070-30-7

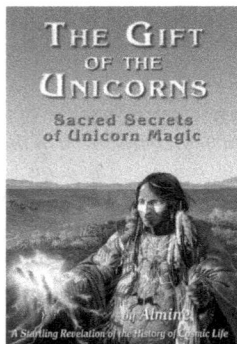

The Gift of the Unicorns *Second Edition*
Sacred Secrets of Unicorn Magic
These life-changing insights into the deep mystical secrets of the earth's past puts the cosmic role of humanity into perspective. It gives meaning to the suffering of the ages and solutions of hope and predicts the restoration of white magic. An enlightening explanation of the causes of the Great Fall and our ascent out of ages of forgetfulness into a remembrance of our divine new purpose and oneness, is masterfully given. Truly an inspiring book!

Published: 2009, 284 pages, soft cover, 6 x 9, ISBN: 978-1-934070-29-1

Other books by Almine

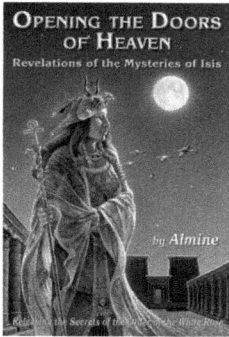

Opening the Doors of Heaven *Second Edition*
Revelations of the Mysteries of Isis
Through a time-travel tunnel, linking Ireland and Egypt, Isis sent a small group of masters to prepare for the day when her mysteries would once again be released to the world to restore balance and enhance life.

They established the Order of the White Rose to guard the sacred objects and the secrets of Isis. In an unprecedented event heralding the advent of a time of light, these mysteries are released for the first time.

Published: 2009, 312 pages, soft cover, 6 x 9 ISBN: 978-1-934070-31-4

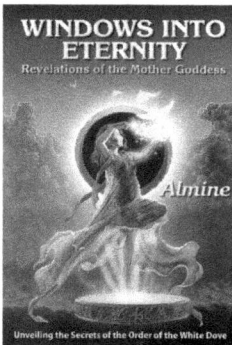

Windows Into Eternity *Second Edition*
Revelations of the Mother Goddess
This book provides unparalled insight into ancient mysteries. Almine, an internationally recognized mystic and teacher, reveals the hidden laws of existence. Transcending reason, delivering visionary expansion, this metaphysical masterpiece explores the origins of life as recorded in the Holy Libraries.
The release of information from these ancient libraries is a priceless gift to humankind. The illusions found in the building blocks of existence are exposed, as are the purposes of Creation.

Published: 2009, 320 pages, soft cover, 6 x 9, ISBN: 978-1-934070-32-1

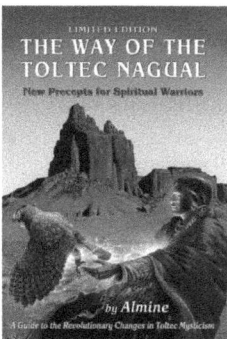

The Way of the Toltec Nagual
New Precepts for the Spiritual Warrior
Not only is this wisdom packed book a guide for serious students of the Toltec way, but also a font of knowledge for all truth-seekers. Mapping out the revolutionary changes in Toltec mysticism, it presents the precepts of mastery sought out by all who travel the road of illumination and spiritual warriorship. Almine reveals publicly for the first time, the ancient power symbols used by Toltec Naguals to assist in obtaining freedom from illusion. Bonus section: Learn about the hidden planets used by Toltecs and the Astrology of Isis.

Published: 2009, 240 pages, soft cover, 6 x 9, ISBN: 978-1-934070-56-7

CDs by Almine

Each powerful presentation has a unique musical background unaltered as channeled from Source.
Truly a work of art.

The Power of Silence
Few teaching methods empty the mind, but rather fill it with more information. As one who has achieved this state of silence, Almine meticulously maps out the path that leads to this state of expanded awareness.

The Power of Self-Reliance
Cultivating self-reliance is explained as resulting from balancing the sub-personalities—key components to emotional autonomy.

Mystical Keys to Ascended Mastery
The way to overcome and transcend mortal boundaries is clearly mapped out for the sincere truth seeker.

The Power of Forgiveness
Digressing from traditional views that forgives a perceived injury, this explains the innocence of all experience. Instead of showing how to forgive a wrong, it acknowledges wholeness.

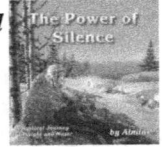

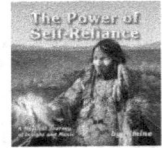

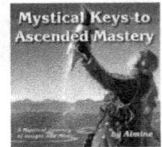

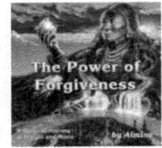

Visit Almine's websites:

www.astrology-of-isis.com

www.arubafirina.com

www.ascensionangels.com

www.alminehealing.com

www.ascendedmastery.com

www.lifeofmiracles.com

www.mysticalkingdoms.com

www.earthwisdomchronicles.com

www.divinearchitect.com

www.incorruptiblewhitemagic.com

www.wheelsofthegoddess.com

www.ancientshamanism.com

www.wayofthetoltecnagual.com

www.schoolofarcana.org

www.belvaspata.org

Diary: www.alminediary.com

www.spiritual-healing-for-animals.com

Visit Almine's website **www.spiritualjourneys.com** for workshop locations and dates, take an online workshop, listen to an internet radio show, or watch a video. Order one of Almine's many books, CD's, or an instant download.

Phone Number: 1-877-552-5646

www.ingramcontent.com/pod-product-compliance
Lightning Source LLC
Chambersburg PA
CBHW070928270326
41927CB00011B/2776